DANCE FITNESS

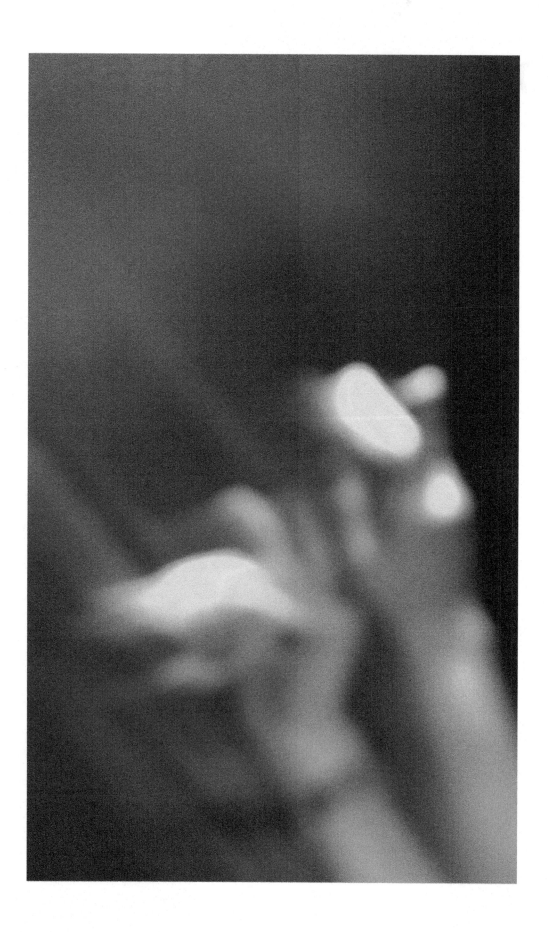

Marina Aagaard

DANCE FITNESS

Fitness dance
– latin, funk and dance group exercise

aagaard

DANCE FITNESS
Fitness dance – latin, funk and dance group exercise

Copyright © 2014 Marina Aagaard

First Edition.

ISBN 978-87-92693-73-0

Cover photo: Photos:	istock.com © A. EropoB s. 2, Kat Jackson ©, s. 12, Gerrit Prenger ©, s. 8, 166 © Aalborg Sportshøjskole, s. 20, sxc.hu © Mateusz Atroszko, s. 30, DJJensen s. 40, Bartlomiej Stroinski, www.stroinski.pl. © s. 51, Claus Petersen © CPHotography, s. 57, Microsoft clip art, s. 72, freeimages @ Michal Zacharzewski s. 8, 102-162, 172, Henrik Elstrup s. 68, 164; Leif Nygaard ©
Cover design, text and drawings:	Marina Aagaard
Printing:	Lulu, USA

No book can replace the services of a physician, exercise physiologist or other qualified health or exercise professionel.
The programs and exercises in this book may not be for everyone.
Any application of the information set forth in the following pages is at the reader's discretion and sole risk.

Marina Aagaard
www.marinaaagaardblog.com
www.fitnesswellnessworld.com

PREFACE

DANCE FITNESS
Fitness dance – latin, funk and dance group exercise
is about dance fitness moves and methods for group
exercise instructors, who want to develop and progress
dance workouts.

Dancing in fitness, for fun and health, has had a great
revival during latter years.
Lots of exercisers are experiencing first hand, that dance
exercise is a fantastic way to get into shape.
It is enjoyable, does not feel like hard work and provides
visible results even with a moderate effort.
Fitness dancers can improve stamina, coordination and
balance and burn fat, if the right methods are used.

Unfortunately, however, a great many exercisers find, that
dancing is hard or difficult, and more than a few experience knee problems, when dancing.
Frustration and overuse injuries can be avoided in almost
all cases, when the instructor picks the right steps and
progressions for the target group and teaches how to
move in a motivating way.

This book provides the prerequisites for accomplishing
just that. The information is based on 30 years of fitness
and dancing as well as sports research.
The aim is to inspire group exercise instructors to have
even more fun and success with dance fitness.

Marina Aagaard, *Master of Fitness and Exercise*

CONTENT

CONTENT

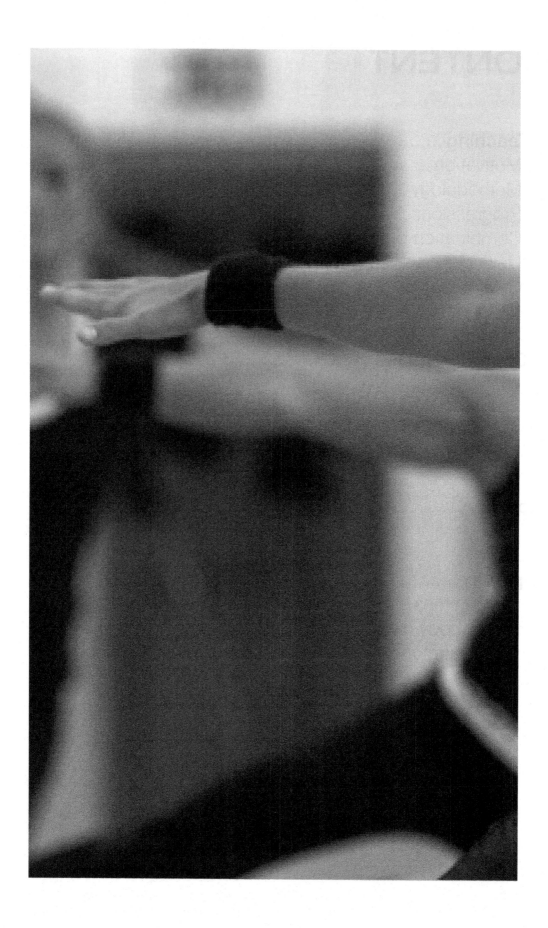

Chapter 1 | **Introduction**

Dance fitness is about dance in a fitness context. It is dedicated to teachers and instructors in group exercise teaching various forms of dance fitness to different target groups. The book covers dance fitness movements as well as succesful dance fitness group instruction.

The goal is to inspire; to 1) present all the tools for creating more motivating choreography for improved cardiovascular health and coordination and 2) provide diverse ideas for designing and teaching dance fitness classes for dance fitness exercisers at different levels.

Happy reading and dancing

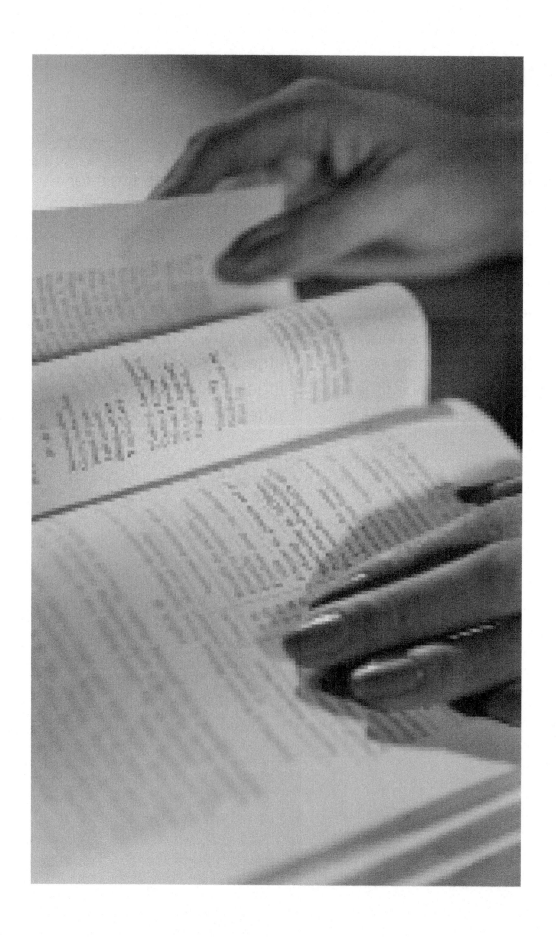

Chapter 2 | **Basics**

Dance Fitness group exercise comes in many styles with latin, funk and powerdance being some of the most popular.

ZumbaFitness is based on easy steps performed to latin music and popular dance music.
Other concepts include Batuka and the Groove Method, 'free' dance.

The difference between dance fitness and most traditionel dance is, that in fitness exercises want a cardio workout and fatburning – apart from fun and performance.

Dance fitness styles differ from club to club, so instructors have many options with regard to the dance class design ...

... a chance to give the class a personal touch; of course respecting the general class description given in the schedule of the fitness centre or club.

Dance Fitness benefits

- **Cardiovascular fitness**
  – and fatburning

- **Strength-endurance**
  – depending on the chosen exercises

- **Flexibility**
  Active and passive, static and dynamic

- **Coordination**
  Rhythm
  Arm-leg coordination
  Eye-hand-or-foot
    coordination
  Spacial awareness
  Balance, static and
    dynamic stability

Better dance fitness – like this!

Dance is fun, it brings happiness and joy, and improves cardiovascular fitness and coordination without seeming like an exhausting workout.

Still dance or rather dance instruction is 'feared' by some group exercise instructors;

*"It is difficult", "It is not for my body", "The exercisers cannot do the steps",
"I can't integrate dance steps in my classes" or
"It is too complicated"...*

It *may* feel challenging if you have to follow the moves of another dance instructor giving a master class or advanced class in a style you are not used to. However, when *you* are the instructor in control of the moves, the style and the rate of progression ... then it is quite easy.

Dance fitness is 'freestyle' steps and movements according to your own rules ...

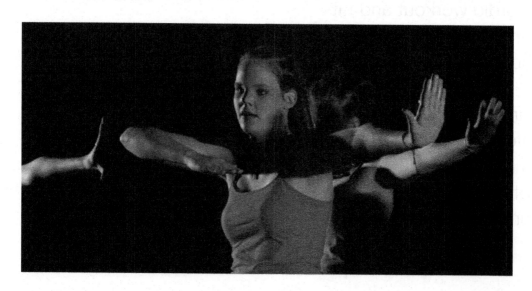

Better dance fitness – like this!

Everybody can dance!

Instructors can; when they observe and learn; watch MTV, watch music- and dance videos and -shows, attend hip-hop, salsa or modern dance classes and workshops and *practice; dance, dance, dance.*

Participants can; when they have the right dance conditions:
Great music and moves and proficient instruction; e.g. timely cueing and counting and peptalk.

In dance the music and the body is used more intensely than in other cardiovascular workouts, so it requires some practice, if you are new to it. As a bonus you improve bodily awareness and control and have a more balanced workout.

You can make dance fitness classes even more enjoyable – with optimal effect and minimal risc of injury – like this:

"Great dancers are not great because of their technique; they are great because of their passion."
Martha Graham (1894-1991)

Better dance fitness – like this!

Music Dancing requires the right original music, not mainstream pop, pitched up or down. Use latin music for latin, hip-hop for funk, etc.

Structure Dance fitness should be structured like other group exercise classes with warm-up, cardio (dance), cooldown and stretching. Often resistance training is left out; it is not quite in sync with dance music and mood.

Warm-up A warm-up of 7-10 minutes is a must. The easier and more gradual the start, the better the workout and learning process. Do a balanced mix of (right/left) exercises.

Dance Lots of rhythm: Mix slow and fast moves. Add upper body moves with style. It does not have to be difficult to look good. Use all of the room, fill it up with dance.

Asymmetry In many classes the same block, series, is performed with both a right and left lead. Bodily wise, but all too predictable. (Also) plan for asymmetrical blocks, but balance left and right lead steps for balanced workouts, that feels good during and after class.

Organisation Perform choreography close together as a team, in to or more groups or in pairs. This adds a touch of real 'show dance' ...

Better dance fitness – like this!

Lead leg   Starting with a left food lead is dance-specific and o.k. However, in most group exercise classes you start with a right foot lead; this makes exercisers feel 'at home'.

Cooldown   If you have been working hard, you should have a cooldown of 3-5 minutes to lower your heart rate gradually. It is healthy, feels good and is a nice transition into stretching.

Stretching   Dance fitness classes finishes with stretching, static, held, stretches. Work on balance and flexibility with progressive stretches, so the exercisers become more flexible; having full range of motion makes dancing easier.

Style   *Attitude!* Dance with body language – express yourself.

Outfit   Shoes should have low friction, so turns are easy to perform. They should also be flexible without too much sole.
Bare feet are also an option, but this can be hard on the feet, when doing runs, jumps and (hip-)hop.

Loose fitting clothes make many movements look more 'dancing'.
Tight fitting clothes are better for showing exactly how the moves should be done.

Better dance fitness – like this!

Contraindicated exercises

Dance fitness is for (almost) everyone; children, youth, adults, seniors and the elderly – as long as the dance is adapted to suit the target group.
Some dance activities, however, are not optimal for:
Pregnant women*; because of the risk of falling or twisting a knee.* ***People with knee problems****; because of the turns and twists. First do basic training for knee strength.*

Dance is fun and healthy, however, there are elements of risk; you need to protect the knees. In many dances a certain level of strength and flexibility is needed for control.

Risky moments, especially for beginners and people with knee problems or overweight, are:

- **Twists, piruettes and turns**; they can be hard on the knees and requires concentration and muscle control.

- **Rotation of the legs**, the femur (thigh bone) should rotate at the hip *without* knee rotation; this movement can be difficult to master initially.

- **Lunges and sidelunges**, large steps forward or outward.

- **Sudden movements**, fast steps and direction changes.

- **Jumps and leaps**; may also be hard on the back.

Better dance fitness – like this!

Contraindicated exercises – continued

In dance fitness you should apply general safety precautions, eg. not bend the knees maximally during difficult exercises and not hyperextend the back (excessively). This is advisable, as recreational dance exercisers often do not have the strength or dance technique to control the body in the end ranges of motion.
In dance for skilled dancers you can dance away with full range of motion and total body movements.

In dance fitness you can still do most movements with your body, though, depending on fitness level and health.

Is it o.k. to bend the knees more than 90 degrees?
Yes, of course. They are designed for that, also during squats and lunges. However, with control and knees and feet should be aligned. *Do not twist your knees!*

Is it o.k. to extend knees and elbows completely?
Yes, include full range of motion for better performance; better stretches and strength. E.g. if your knees are always bent, you are not stretching your hamstrings.
Do not hyperextend or lock your joints.

Is it o.k. to lower your head below heart level?
Yes, of course, if you have a 'normal' healthy body.
In general: If you have had your head down for a period of time, get up slowly, so you don't feel dizzy.

AVOID KNEE PROBLEMS

Unfortunately quite many recreational dancers experience knee problems, when attending dance classes. So:

It is **very important**, that dance fitness instructors point out, that *"dancing is a super workout, but it is imperative, that you are 'on your toes' when turning, keep knees and feet aligned, and **do not** twist the knees".* Also offer help and advice: *"If you do experience knee problems, tell me and I will find an alternative exercise or variation – you can and should dance without knee pain."*

Remind participants to wear shoes with low friction or dance in bare feet.
And to pay special attention, whenever they are twisting and turning.

Better dance fitness – like this!

Avoid injuries

To avoid falls, acute injuries, overuse injuries and extreme muscle soreness during dance fitness, the instructor should take certain safety precautions, when putting together the choreography and when teaching:

- Adapt the choreography to the desired level; the level is described on the club homepage or in class flyers.

- At the beginning of the class tell participants, that dance fitness requires, that you are in control of your feet and knees, so you should progress at your own pace and avoid doing too much too soon.

- Inform exercisers about alternatives if necessary.

- Work on stability and technique, gradual progression, before moving on to more advanced moves; pivots and turns within 1-2 beats are advanced moves.

- Differentiate the moves during class, give options for beginning, intermediate and advanced level.

- Use gradual progression and adapt exercises, so that most of the exercisers can follow (most of the time).

- Use clear precise cueing at the right time, in advance, so exercisers know, when to travel or change moves.

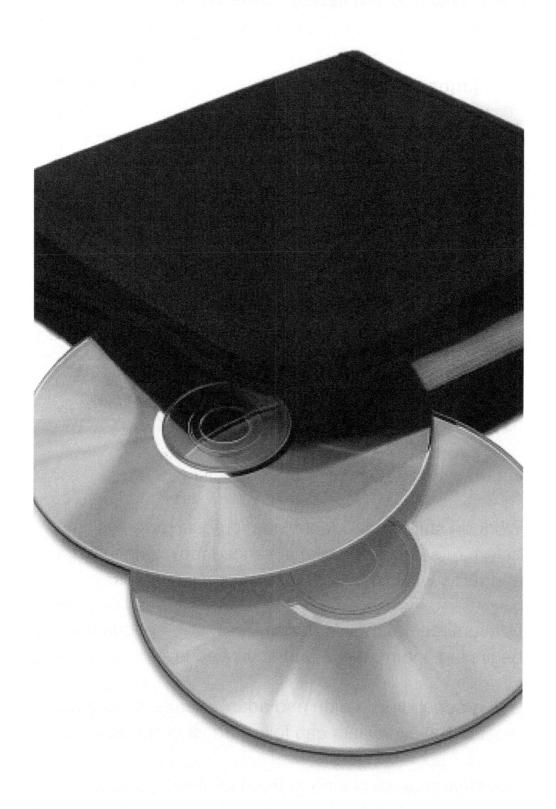

Chapter 3 | **Music**

A great dance fitness experience is dependent on good music. Using the right genre and harmonies sets the mood. Music provides inspiration for creating exciting choreography and makes dance fitness even more motivating. Knowledge of music and structure makes it easier to use the music optimally.

Genres and music selection

There are more than a hundred different music genres. Dance fitness music is often jazz, r'n'b, lounge, house, latin, etc. Music for group exercise, including funk and latin is available as mixes; either re-mixed or cover versions in long mixes of 55-75 minutes of duration.

The advantage of a mix is its steady rhythm and regular structure, often with four beats per measure throughout the mix. This makes it easy to use the music without prior analysis or counting beats; you can just put on the music and start teaching right away. The disadvantage is, that one does not have the same 'feeling' in music with a (heavy) base rhythm added, and in a mix you seldom like every song. The advantage of finding your own music is getting original songs in your own taste, whether it is found on CDs, downloaded. or streamed. The disadvantage may be an irregular structure or unexpected changes in the music, which demands more pre-class preparation.

Beats and bars

Music has a rhythm consisting of a pulse or **beats.** These are grouped into **measures** structuring the music into segments of a given number of beats. The measure is also often referred to as a '**bar**'.

The number of beats in a measure is defined by the top number in the time signature of the music, e.g. *2/4 for polka, 3/4 for the waltz or 4/4 in pop music.* In the polka each measure therefore has two beats, and one counts 1-2, 1-2, 1-2. In the 3-beat measure of the waltz one counts 1-2-3, 1-2-3, where as measures of four beats is common in pop music, counting 1-2-3-4, 1-2-3-4.

The time signature, 2/4, 3/4 or 4/4, is found by counting the number of beats within the measure.

Start by counting the first beat, which is often accented, then counting the following beats, until reaching the first accented beat of the next measure.

Two 4/4-measures very often corresponds to one verse line; in group exercise, dance fitness, this is called an 'eight-count' (phrase).
Here one would count to eight, even if there is a marked beat on '5', the first beat of the next 4/4-measure.
Four eight-counts form a 32-count/4-phrase block; a perfect match for a pop music verse or chorus.

Note: Some original music has passages with 2, 4, 8 or 12 beats. Be aware of this and have the right number of steps to match the music.

In most group exercise music beats are heavily accentuated with hardly any difference in accent:

Beat accent	**I**	**I**	**I**	**I**	**I**	**I**	**I**	**I**
Beat # (2 measures)	1.	2.	3.	4.	1.	2.	3.	4.
Count (dance fitness)	1.	2.	3.	4.	5.	6.	7.	8.

Other music has a more nuanced accentuation:

Beat accent	**I**	I	**I**	I	**I**	I	**I**	I
Beat # (2 measures)	1.	2.	3.	4.	1.	2.	3.	4.
Count (fitness dance)	1.	2.	3.	4.	5.	6.	7.	8.

Here the beats on odd counts are accented, often markedly on the first and 'fifth' beat. Even beats are often less marked. Accented beats are '**down-beat**', unaccented beats are called '**up-beat**'.

If you move between the beats of the base rhythm, this is called '**off-beat**'. This is seen in funk with **syncopated** moves, moves 'off' the base rhythm.
Example: 1-*and*-2, 3-*and*-4 or -*and*-1-*and*- 2, -*and*-3-*and* 4.

Up-Beat		2.		4.		6.		8.
Base rhythm	**I** -I	- **I**	- I	- **I**	-I	- **I**	- I
Down-Beat	1.		3.		5.		7.	
Off-Beat	-and- -and- -and- -and- -and- -and- -and-

Musical structure

Music is composed of several elements, which form its structure (example page 75).
For creating a good choreography the main structure of the music has to be found, for example:

Intro	Introduction, 32 beats, 4-8+ eights
Verse (A)	Tells a story, 4 x 8 beats, four verse lines
Chorus (B)	Refrain, the part of the song, you remember and sing along to
Bridge (C)	A part for variation, contrast or transition
Outro (coda)	Ending; in a mix often 'hidden' in the transition into the next song

When composing choreography, the number of steps should fit the music structure, e.g. 4 x 8 beats:

Right (32 beats total)
1. 1 x 8   Chassé 4 front
2. 1 x 8   Touch out 4
3. 1 x 8   Slide 4 back
4. 1 x 8   Kneelift 4

Wrong (52 beats total)
Walk 4 forward (4 beats)
Touch out 8 (16 beats)
Slide 8 back (16 beats)
Kneelift 8 (16 beats)

As almost all pop music verses and refrains are 4 x 8 beats, the choreography should match this, so music and movements are in harmony. Dance fitness choreography is mostly composed of 'blocks' of 4 x 8 beats for either block choreography or verse-chorus choreography.

Phrase

It is not only essential to follow the beat, it is of equal importance to follow the phrases of the music.

A phrase is a musical sentence.

In group exercise a phrase corresponds to a line in a verse or chorus, an '**eight-count**' (2x4), where as in classical music it can be anything from a few melodic notes to many bars of music joined together.

When dancing the combinations must start in time with the first beat in the eight-count, the start of the phrase. Movements are easier to perform and feel more natural, when you follow the phrases.

Note: If the instructor by mistake starts out of sync with the line of the verse, e.g. on the 'third' beat, this will feel awkward. Especially dancers, who are used to moving to music, will find it difficult to follow.

Four 'eight-counts' is a block

Example: Block choreography for one verse:

1. 1 x 8   Walk 8 forward, walk low with bent legs, feet cross.
2. 1 x 8   Stand, twist on the spot R, L, R2, L, R, L2.
3. 1 x 8   Stomp back 4, big steps, double stomps.
4. 1 x 8   Jack in/cross legs (1), jack out (2). 4x.

Tempo

The music tempo affects the mood; inspires to run, jog or walk. Tempo also influences exercise selection, e.g. in funk you perform syncopated and double tempo moves; this requires music with a slower beat.
The movements can be performed at a slower or faster tempo than the beat, but should be in accordance with the mood and melody of the music.

Below you find a guide to number of beats per minute, bpm, however other tempos may be used as long as the exercises are adapted to the purpose and target group.

Music tempo recommendations	
Activity and movements	Beats per minute
Warm-up	120-135
Walking and dance	100-130
Swinging movements	100-130
Hopping and jumping	120-140
Jogging and running	140-180
Aerobic dance	130-160
Modern dance	100-130+
Jazz dance (r'n'b)	110-130
Cooldown/cardiofunk	110-140
Funk/hip hop	90-120
Total body and swinging movements	60-80
Strength training movements	80-120
Stretching	< 100

Table 3.1: Music tempo guide. You can find the music tempo by counting the number of beats per minute. Clap to the beat and count each clap for a full minute, check www.physicaltunes.com or a DJ homepage or use an app.

Volume

The volume also plays a part in setting the mood. It improves the dance experience, when the music is at a moderate volume initially, then (slightly) higher during the dancing, lower during cooldown and very low during stretching and relaxation.

Warning: Many instructors have lost part of their hearing, without noticing, and are unaware of how loud the music is. Therefore instructors should ask the participants if the volume is o.k. Often the sound level during group exercise classes becomes way too loud, which makes the class less enjoyable, and unhealthy, to attend.

It may be tempting to turn up the volume louder and louder, however, do protect everyone's ears.
In the front of the room, with the back to the speakers, it is difficult to tell how loud it is. So walk around the room, get close to the speakers, and adjust the sound level. Note; your hearing diminishes gradually without you noticing, so be extra careful. Too loud noise may result in tinnitus, a constant ringing in your ears. It is incurable. *Many instructors suffer from tinnitus.*

Click-click-click-click-click-click-click, no thanks! Avoid stress. If you use an mp3-player, then prepare: Have your track-list ready with your songs in the right order. It is stressful and annoying and breaks the flow of the class, when the instructor keeps zapping for songs!

Sound

Quality sound, and sound control, is very important. Unfamiliar with the sound system and loudness? Show up well in advance; perform a sound check. When you perform a sound check, and also right before class, turn the volume to zero. Then gradually turn up the volume to find the right sound level. Adjust the bass and treble levels to be neutral or tuned to improve the sound quality. Often these adjustments are set wrongly, which degrades the music quality. It may be difficult for the instructor to hear if the sound level is right from the front of the room. Walk around the room, also in front of the loudspeakers, to find out how loud it is. Check the microphone for sound; does microphone volume match the music volume.

Microphone technique

- Do not use the microphone as an excuse for turning up the volume louder and louder.

- The microphone must be close to the mouth.

- Set microphone volume at the right level; not too loud, so that it wails.

- Speak in a normal tone, not too loud; never yell directly into the microphone; typical mistake.

- Speak clearly. If you mumble, this is amplified by the microphone.

- Never whistle into the microphone, as this is damaging to the ears.

- Remember, when you are giving individual feedback to a participant; turn off or put the microphone on 'mute'!

Troubleshouting

Sometimes the sound system *"does not work"* ...
If no sound is heard, it is often because:

- The main switch is not turned to on!

- One part of the sound system is not on.

- The plug (main) has been pulled out accidentally.

- The loudspeaker plug has been pulled out.

- The wires between the different parts of the sound system have been pulled out and not been reconnected; a frequent event, when others connect their own PC or mp3-player and forget to reconnect the cables.

- The sound system power is switched on, but there is a loose connection, damaged switch.
  Try turning it off and on again, maybe it works.

- The wiring may be damaged. Gently move the wire or plug to hear if this is the problem. Then get it fixed.

- The ports of the mixer may be damaged; get the sound system checked by a professional.

- The volume dial on the amplifier or mixer, the master or individual volume, is at zero!
  It is true ... this often happens, so do double check before panicking.

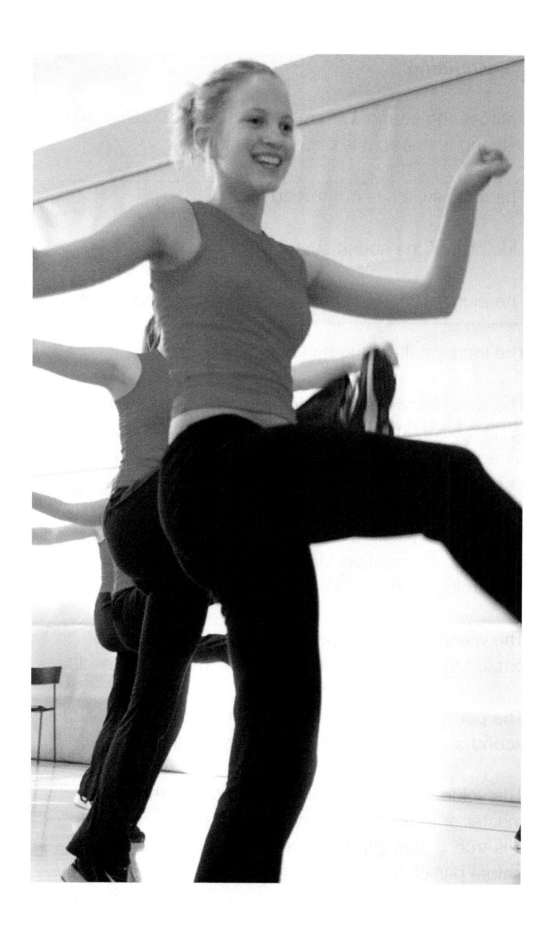

Chapter 4 | **Class design**

Dance fitness classes should be structured like any other group exercise class. The typical class framework is:

- Warm-up
- Dance, cardio
- Cooldown
- Stretching

This framework 1) makes the dance class seem planned, 2) provides a foundation for freestyling and experimenting and 3) ensures that exercisers will enjoy a complete and balanced workout.

The dance fitness class can evolve progressively, building to a 'finale' and ending with a cooldown – or there can be several peaks during class, almost like interval training.

In dance fitness classes the goal is to have a fun and balanced workout with all-round body work, improved cardiovascular fitness and increased fatburning.

This can be achieved by dancing non-stop without rest-pauses.

Structure minimizes stress
Most people are busy in the everyday and have a lot on their minds. By providing a structured, easy to do workout, where exercisers experience familiar activities and doable steps, feelings of stress and lack of control are reduced and chances of an enjoyable workout with feelings of competence are increased.

Dance fitness flow

Keywords in fun, popular dance fitness classes are **flow** and **balance**.

It feels good, when all the moves are linked and the workout flows without interruption; a constant flow from start to finish.

Create a flow experience:

- Have a master plan.

- Prepare and organize, so classes run smooth-ly from the start:

- Have the music ready. Demo and explain special steps.

- Build the moves, the choreography, with flow throughout class.

- Run a non-stop class, eg. no fixed water breaks:
  Make them optional.

At the beginning of class instructors can encourage participants to have water breaks at their own pace, and recommend drinking water during the day and after the class as needed.

Note: Fixed water breaks, up to 4-5 times per class, breaks the flow and are annoying, especially to those participants, who do not wish to drink at that particular time ...

As water is not strictly necessary during shorter workouts, 30-40 minutes of cardio work, these communal water breaks can be left out.

During particularly warm weather, when you sweat a lot, the instructor should, however, remind the participants to drink water regularly.

Dance fitness should be fun, healthy and safe. This is possible with some simple precautions:

1) Select safe moves; avoid or minimize risky steps and exercises.

2) Select specific moves; the exercises should fit the target group and be demoed at different levels.

3) Remind participants to be careful when doing turns, lateral movements and deep knee-bends; watch the knees.

4) Provide technique cues to eliminate poor posture and sloppy, uncontrolled and ballistic movements, hyperextension of joints.

Tip: Limit the amount of technical cues. Give cues in small doses and focus on having fun.

Design enjoyable dance fitness classes with the target group in mind:

Intensity
Intensity should progress from low at the beginning, increase during dancing and decrease at the end of class.

Impact
Beginners do not have the strength for jumps, leaps or deep kneebends. Demo these exercises with smaller range of motion options and low impact alternatives.

Coordination
Difficulty level. Provide variation, keep exercisers moving; it motivates and lessens the risk of injuries; when you are attentive, there is less risk of falling.

Methodology
Use logical progressions, so everybody follows without stress and stops.

Dance fitness class structure

Dance fitness classes can easily be enhanced, when you are familiar with music structure, sound, choreography basics as well as physiology, sports science and psychology.

Design dance fitness classes with aesthetic as well as physical aspects in mind:
1) **Harmony** between music and movements, perfect timing and precise moves.
2) **Proper progressions**, so dancing and exercising feels good, effective and motivating.

The perfect class? Dance fitness instructors can use a general class structure model (table 4.1); this will give some ideas for
1) the overall structure,
2) elements to consider
3) class sequence,
4) duration of parts, and
5 music tempo guidelines for healthy, safe classes. You can then concentrate on the fun stuff; music and movement selection.

The right framework will provide a solid yet flexible danse class foundation.

Avoid rest-pauses
Keep the dance fitness class going. Extended breaks between the songs and dances will lower participant motivation and workout intensity.
This happens, if the instructor spends time looking for songs or gives long-winded explanations.
If you have breaks between songs, then 1) keep the participants moving, 2) make it optional to have waterbreaks and 3) keep eye contact.

DANCE FITNESS CLASS STRUCTURE			
PART	CONTENT	DURATION	MUSIC
Introduction	Welcome. Presentation (start of season and for newcomers). Short intro: Class content.	1-2 min.	0 BPM No music
Warm-up	Easy low impact steps. All-round movements. Dynamic stretches. Intensity progression. Create joy, success.	7-10 min. 1-2 songs	115-135 BPM Low-moderate volume
Cardio Coordi-nation Dance	Dance-based cardio. Low, moderate, and high impact. Fun. Effective. Safe. Difficulty progression. Differentiate moves.	20-40 min. 6-10 songs	100-130+ BPM Moderate-higher volume
Cooldown I	Easy movements; low impact steps. Balance exercises and rhythmic stretches. Intensity regression.	3-10 min. 1-2 songs	100-130 BPM Low-moderate volume
Cooldown II Stretching Relaxation	Stretches, static, hold >15-30 sec. Increase flexibility. Focus on breathing, relaxation and wellness.	5-10 min. 1-2 songs	< 100 BPM Low volume
Outro	Closing. See you! Questions?/Requests?	1-2 min.	0 BPM No music

Table 4.1: Dance Fitness class structure. Aagaard, 2014.

Warm-up

The warm-up is of para-mount importance; it should make participants feel successful and happy. Start basic and progress gradually, so everybody are getting warm and ready, all while feeling confident and energetic.

Warm-ups should include:

- **Rhythmic limbering**
  large muscles working;
  low impact legwork

- **Isolations;**
  specific movements
  for all major joints

- **Rhythmic stretching;**
  movements increasing
  range of motion

Warm-ups should match the activity to follow, so dance fitness warm-ups should include steps and rehearsel moves for the choreography to come.

The warm-up can be structured in a linear way, one thing at a time, with-out (long) combinations, or as block choreography in which the movements are combined to blocks of 4 x 8 counts of music.

The warm-up should include dynamic stretches for the hips and legs and mobility work for the spine and shoulders.

The warm-up should start at a basic level with a gradual increase in both **difficulty, intensity** and **impact**; *superlow, low and moderate impact for warming up.*
No high impact, e.g. hops, during the first 5 minutes!

The participants should get warmed up feeling in control, without having to concentrate or work too hard too soon.

Dance and cardio

Dance fitness has two goals; 1) to dance and have fun and 2) to get in shape; to improve cardiovascular fitness, coordination and body composition.

How? Get the body moving and keep it moving; use a variety of moves for all the major muscles. Some moves may seem small, but when major and minor muscles are working at the same time, the workout gets intense.

In dance you train two fitness aspects at the same time; cardiovascular fitness and coordination, eg. controlling arms and legs and keeping the rhythm and balance. For variety *and* exercise the base moves can be altered and combined almost endlessly.

Tip: When participants are ready, from time to time give them some base moves and encourage some 'freestyling'.

Seven to heaven (Yvonne Lin, YLab)

Increase intensity, energy consumption, via

- Tempo – speed, acceleration and deceleration
- Horisontal travelling – diverse floor patterns
- Vertical 'travelling' – moving up and down
- Load – muscle contraction (and external resistance)
- Amplitude – large movements, full range of motion
- Lever – long lever movements with arms and legs
- Active muscles – more muscles, higher intensity

Cooldown

Following intense activity with the heart rate up, you should gradually lower it to resting level.

This is accomplished with a gradual cooldown right after your dance phase; this is your **cooldown** (I).

A cooldown is essential: Keep moving to ensure, that the muscles keep pumping the blood back to the heart.
If you stop too suddenly, the blood is not pumped efficiently back to the heart and you may feel dizzy or faint.

During the cooldown you apply the principles of the warm-up, but in reverse order:

Gradually reduce the intensitety by going from high to low impact, from travelling to stationary moves and from large to small moves; use slower music and movements.

As part of the cooldown, you can, if time allows, do standing stretches for the muscles of the hips and legs; hip flexors, quads, buttocks and hamstrings as well as calves a.o.

Depending on the class goal and time frame the stretches can be of long or short duration; the stretches are typically held from 15-45 seconds.

Balance exercises can also be included in the cooldown. Either as an integral part of the stretches, e.g. standing hip-flexor stretch on one leg, or as regular balance exercises such as scales, T-balances, or yoga 'trees'.

Stretching

During the last part of class, cooldown II, you should lower the heart rate further and stretch the muscles gently. Increasing or maintaining flexibility makes it easier to move and to dance.

The last part of class is important physically and mentally, because it is the 'final'; it concludes the dance experience and participants remember this last part, so: Stretching should be planned with as much preparation as the other parts of class. And even if the stretching does not have take up a lot of time, it should be presented as valuable and relevant.

Stretching should feel good (not painful). Stretching should be felt as a firm pull on the belly of the muscle.

Pain in tendons and joints is not healthy stretching and should be avoided.

During the final cooldown use static stretches; for the tight muscles; calves, shin muscles, hamstrings, quads, hip flexors, buttocks and adductors. If you have time, stretch smaller muscles, too. All-round stretching feels good and promotes relaxation and well-being.

In dance (fitness) it is beneficial, functional, to include longer stretches to increase flexibility, eg. 30-60+ seconds. Focus on deep breathing through the nose as this facilitates relaxation.

Tip: For extra flexibility, required in certain dances, warm-up thoroughly and hold stretches for 2-5 min.

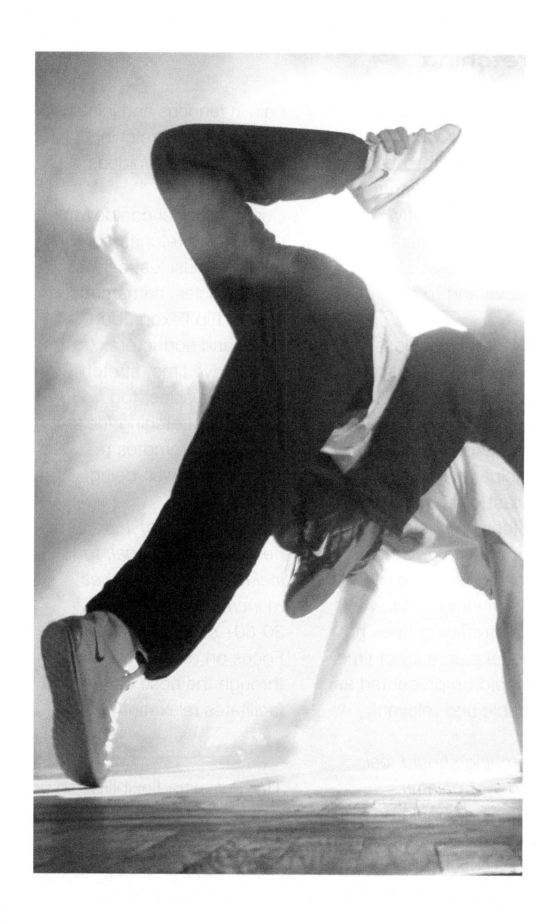

40

Chapter 5 | **Choreography**

Choreography is about composing, merging and styling movements.
Dance fitness choreography is based on music and base moves, which are styled with variations and combinations for exercise or performance purposes.

Listen to the chosen music; first **intuitively**, to sense, which moves are suitable, then **analytically**, so you establish the structure of the music, verse, chorus and interlude and number of beats per minute.

Group exercise instructors normally create blocks of choreography as they go along without prior music analysis. This is fine for fitness and saves time, but requires knowledge of music structure and a large repertoire of exercises.

Choreography can be composed intuitively without considering workout (physiological) outcome.
In dance fitness, however, for best results, you often create choreography from base moves and develop the dances systematically.

When using a model or a framework it is easy to get started and create fun, motivating choreography.

The foundation of dance fitness are dance steps based on basic steps (page 45) used in group exercise classes, but stylized for a new, eg. funky or latin, look.
The simpler the basic steps, the easier it is to create new steps and moves ... instead of the same old step touches, V-steps and grapevines!

Styles

All steps, combinations and upper body movements can be mixed and matched in different ways.

The common methods of creating choreography in group exercise, aerobic gymnastics and show routines are:

Block

Block choreography is built by blocks, parts, of 4 x 8 counts of choreography. This is the preferred method in group exercise and the easiest method to plan and teach.

Block choreography can be composed in advance or developed during the class without preparation.

In group exercise classes, there are normally 3-4 blocks of choreography depending on class duration and level.

Verse/chorus

This is the foundation of *concept training*; fixed three month programs, eg. Les Mills' BodyAttack, Zumba Fitness a.o.

The choreography is based on an analysis of the music structure; you identify the verses, choruses and bridges.

Each part is given its own steps and exercises; a block of choreography for every verse and a one for the chorus; every time the chorus is repeated, that block of choreography is repeated.

Base

Base choreography has a base of two eight-counts, each with a set of basic steps, e.g. eight jogs and four jacks. This base is progressively made more and more complex.

Base choreography uses the *layering* principle; to put layers on top of the base choreography, eg. direction, travelling etc. As you are not adding more eight-counts, just changing the original 2 x 8, it is an easy way to teach complex choreography. In the end you can add 2 x 8 (e.g. a balance) for a complete block og 4 x 8.

Freestyle

As the name implies 'free style' or improvisation. Freestyle choreography with steps, moves and short combinations is created spontaneously by the instructor and/or participants; it flows freely without being combined into a longer, complex choreography.

Freestyle requires that the instructor has an extensive repertoire of exercises and fairly skilled participants, so the class keeps going.

Show

Show choreography is choreography for shows or performances as in aerobic gymnastics and fitness routines.
You analyze a piece of music from start to finish. Often you need to listen to it a great number of times to identify the exact number of beats, structure and instrumentation.

You make notes of the number and 'position' of beats, measures and phrases and mark vocal and instrumental parts and sound effects.

The music does not need to have perfect eight-counts; it may be more interesting, if the music has an irregular structure.

Following music analyzis, you compose the choreography beat by beat and phrase by phrase, so it fits the music perfectly.

Base moves

The basis for composing dance choreography is the natural movements of the body; ask yourself:

How does the body move?

Walk, run, hop, leap, jump, balance, roll, crawl, climb, swing, pull, push, stretch, bend, twist, turn, etc.

Simple or complex movements:

- **Torso and core movements** (and posture)
  Bend, extend, sidebend right/left, rotate right/left.

- **Lower body movements**
  Bend, extend, abduct, adduct, rotate inwards/outwards.

  Basic lower body motor skills:

Walk	Transfer weight from foot to foot, not airborne
Run	Transfer weight from foot to foot, airborne
Leap	Take off from one foot, land on one or two feet
Jump	Take off from both feet, land on one or two feet

  Include all basic steps (p. 45) – *march (walk), jog (run) and leap and hop on one foot, skip, kneelift, kick, jack and jump (hop), lunge* – and add style according to the music; latin, funk, world music, classical.

- **Upper movements**
  Bend, extend, abduct, adduct, rotate in and out.

FITNESS DANCE | AEROBIC (GYM) BASIC STEPS

STEP	TECHNIQUE/PERFORMANCE	
1 March Walk	• Legs in front: Hip- and kneeflexion. • Controlled ankle movement, toe-ball-heel. • Movements is upwards, not downwards. • Controlled movement; no unwanted movement forward and backward or downward.	
2 Jog Run	• Lower leg maximally back, heel to buttocks: Hip extension. Knee flexion. Knee by or behind opposite knee. Foot plantarflexed in top position. • Controlled ankle movement; toe-ball-heel.	
3 Skip	• Skip starts as a jog, heel to buttocks, then low skip with knee extension. • Controlled movement; the lower leg movement is stopped by the thigh contracting.	
4 Kneelift	• Working leg lifts; hip- and knee flexion, minimum 90 degree hip flexion. • When the thigh is in top position, the lower leg is vertical and the ankle plantarflexed. • The ankle may be dorsiflexed, with control.	
5 Kick	• High kick; hip flexion only, the knee is straight, extended, up and down. The ankle is plantarflexed, foot pointed. Support leg knee bends only slightly.	
6 Jumping jack	• Jump out and in, knees bend. • Natural outward hip rotation. • Controlled take-off and landing, all of foot. • Controlled ankle movement; toe-ball-heel. • Landing; feet together, toes forward or out..	
7 Lunge	• Feet are parallel, together or hip-width apart. • One leg back; hip extension, no rotation. • Heel is lowered to the ground with control. • Low impact: Full body lean, straight line. • High impact: Legs scissors, front and back. The bodyweight is evenly distributed between both feet.	

Figure 5.1: Basic steps in fitness and AER gymnastics, Lin 1994, Aagaard, 2000.

Basic movements

The basic movements can be varied endlessly by changes in the following areas:

- **Coordination**
  Difficulty; easy, intermediate, advanced (complex)

- **Intensity**
  Cardiovascular effect; low, medium or high

- **Impact**
  Reaction force; 'load' on bones and joints;
  non, super low, low, moderate, high, super high

Variation enhances enjoyment and motivation and provides for positive training results; improved health, fitness and performance; e.g.

- better balance
- improved endurance
- Increased flexibilty
- stronger bones and joints

Tip:
When selecting dance fitness movements: Consider the goal of the class, the class description, what is promised in advance, and the health and fitness of the target group. Choose appropriate exercises; consider coordination, intensity and impact. This increases participant motivation and minimizes the risk of injuries.

Base moves

In gymnastics and dance the character of the movements is often described as sustained, swinging or percussive. These expressions are seldom used in dance fitness, but they may inspire dance fitness instructors to focus even more on matching the moves to the music:

Sustained
Continuous movements without interruption. Movements, which are even, steady, prolonged and slow. No sudden stops and starts. Music: New age music and other music without marked accentuations.

Swinging
Swinging, swaying movements, from contract to relax. Initiation of movements and allowing your body or limbs to give in to gravity on the downward phase. Music: Many genres, e.g. jazz and pop.

Percussive
Strong, quick, jerky, sharp movements like punches, pushes, throws, kicks and hops. Music: Many genres with a marked rhythm, e.g. disco, rock and drum'n'bass.

Laban's principles
Dancers use the principles and terminology of Laban (Rudolf Laban, 1879-1958): On the next two pages there is a short summary of his terminology for movement analysis to provide instructors with some ideas for developing more intricate dance fitness choreography.

LABAN QUALITIES OF MOVEMENT		
Quality	Effort quality (contrast)	
SPACE	Direct	Straight, focus directly on the target, limited use of space.
	Flexible	Plastic, curved, elastic, undulating, extended use of space
TIME	Slow	Smooth, hesitant, quiet
	Fast	Sudden, quick, sharp, staccato, excited, hasty, lively, stressful, happy
WEIGHT	Light	Relaxed, caressing, floating, upwards.
	Firm	Heavy, strong, powerful, downwards
FLOW	Bound	Controllered, thoughtful, prepared, stoppable
	Free	Ongoing, continuous, unstoppable.

Table 5.1: Laban movement qualities.

LABAN ACTIONS OF THE BODY			
Basic action	Space	Weight	Time
Stab – push, lunge	straight	firm	quick
Whip – flail, dash	curved	firm	quick
Glide – slip, slide	straight	light	slow
Float – drift, flow	curved	light	slow
Press – push, force	straight	firm	slow
Wring – crunch, squeeze	curved	firm	slow
Hack – chop, strike, clap	straight	light	quick
Waive – flutter, flit	curved	light	quick

Table 5.2: Laban basic action examples.

LABAN MOVEMENTS

SPACE	Personal space	Direction	Up, down, left, right, forward, backward, diagonally
		Shape	Large, small, long, wide, symmetrical, asymmetrical, etc.
		Relation-ship (to objects or people)	Leading/following, meeting/parting, copying/mirroring, unison/canon, question/answer
	General space	Travel	Straight or curved, waves, circles, zig zag, etc.
		Level	High Medium Low
		Plane	Frontal (to the side) Horisontal Sagittal (forward/backward)
TIME	Fast, slow, accelerating, decelerating, sudden, sustained, starting, stopping, etc.		
WEIGHT	Firm. Forceful. Light. Relaxed.		

Table 5.3: Laban movement examples.

Table 5.1, 5.2 and 5.3 show Rudolf Laban (1879-1958) terminolgy in short.

These Laban principles is a unique inspirational tool for creating (advanced) choreography.

Base position

In dance you see all shapes, body positions. There is no right or wrong; not one optimal posture, because it depends on the dance; should you contract or relax, stand tall or crouch?

In basic training, however, walking and balancing, e.g. turns and pirouettes, an upright erect posture and focused gaze is preferable.

Posture check:

From the front
Image a plumb line in front of the centre of the body. Around this line, the torso, hips and shoulders should form a symmetrical image.

From the side
Image a plumb line, passing through the ear, shoulder, hip, knee and ankle joint.

Positions
In ballet there are five basic positions with straight legs. The position of the feet is show here:

1. position. Heels together.

2. position. Heels, feet, apart.

3. position. One foot in front of the other, ankles touch.

4. position. One foot in front of the other, feet apart.

5. position. Feet right in front of each other, together.

Starting position

- Legs together or hip- or shoulder-width apart.

- Feet forward or natural outward rotation.

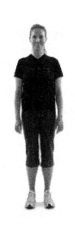

- Knees and feet aligned.

- Knees relaxed, not bent or locked.

- Pelvis in neutral position,
  abs and buttocks stabilize.

- Contract the core to stabilize when needed.

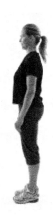

- Spine in neutral position, normal curve.

- Shoulder blades in neutral, not forward.

- Shoulders relaxed and level.

- Neck in neutral position.

> *"Make the impossible possible, the possible easy and the easy elegant."*
>
> Moshe Feldenkrais (1904-1984)

Variations

A very easy method for composing dance fitness choreography, is this:

Use a mix of all the 'raw' basic steps (p. 45) and add one or more of the following seven variations:

- Tempo
- Rhythm
- Direction
- Travelling
- Planes
- Joint movements
- Active muscles

Another method is to use the Laban principles (p. 48-49), which is used extensively in dance and gymnastics.

Laban's principles covers the above variations – with special attention to the quality of movements.

Variations affect the level of difficulty in the dance fitness class.
The more variations, the more complex, difficult, the choreography.

Dance fitness instructors can choose to have many variations, even in beginners' classes ...
but one step at a time, not all variations at the same time or in the same series of steps. Also for beginners the tempo has to be somewhat slower.

Note: *Choreography does not have to be difficult or detailed to look and feel exciting*.
Harmony between music and movements is of primary importance
– and using different rhythms and unexpected or unique movements.

Speed

Music tempo in dance is around 120-140 beats per minute, BPM.
Depending on the genre the tempo can be either faster or slower.

Note: Movement tempo can be the same as or different from music tempo, e.g. half or double tempo.

Perform fast or double tempo movements to increase complexity; this requires a high degree of coordination.

Breaks can make the choreography even more interesting; sudden stops are great for 'agility' training, while longer 'stops' works well for balances.

Note: The heart rate drops quickly during slow movements and balances. Limit these, if the goal is cardiovascular fitness.

Rhythm

All movements can be stylized with different rhythms. E.g. combining steps in half tempo, a tempo and double tempo, e.g. walk slow 1 (1,2) and a tempo 2 (3,4) or maybe syncopated, between beats, on '1-and-2-and'. Or:

Alternating rhythms as in samba (1 -and-2, 3, 4), mambo (1, 2, 3 -and-4), cha-cha (1, 2, 3-and, 4) or waltz 1,2,3 1,2,3 ... include a pause on 7,8, when using pop music, to stay in time with the 'eight-counts'.

Arms, legs and torso can move in different rhythms, which creates variation and increases complexity.

Another kind of rhythm variation is *repeaters;* e.g. a kneelift with the kneelift repeated 2 or more times.

Direction

Direction is the direction of the body in the room, the way you are facing:

Forward, left, right, backward, diagonally and all the positions in between – and combined as in turns.

Direction changes, turns, pivots and pirouettes, dynamic balances, are great for balance work.

Turns can be integrated in the choreography or used as *transitions*, between different parts of the choreography.

Turns are typically ¼, ½, ¾ and 1/1 turn to the left or the right.

1½, 2/1, 3/1 or more turns are mainly seen in advanced dance and for shows and competitions.

Figure 5.2: Basic directions of the body (there are many more). These can be combined with travelling for increased complexity, e.g. walking forward while doing a full turn.

Displacement

Movement of the body's centre of mass up and down or in different directions on the floor.

Vertical displacement is movement of the body up and down; low, medium and high level.

Horizontal displacement, *travelling*, is movement in the horisontal plane, floor patterns:

Forward, backward, sideways right and left, diagonally, circular or patterns; triangles, squares, circles, semicircles, letters (as in Bokwa) or 'freestyle'.

Tip: Think of the room as a three-dimensional box to be filled with movements in all directions and levels. This makes the choreography diverse, dynamic and interesting.

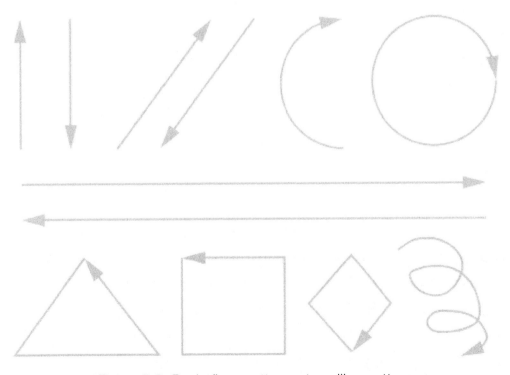

Figure 5.3: Basic floor patterns, travelling patterns.

Planes

The arms and legs can move in different planes. Movement planes are:

- **Frontal plane**
  Sideways, to the side

- **Sagittal plane**
  Forward/backward

- **Transversal plane**
  Horizontal plane

The choreography can be composed to challenge coordination, e.g. moves with the arms and legs in different planes, as in kicking the legs forward, while abducting the arms to the side.

Joint movements

The body moves with various joint movements:

Flexion, extension, abduction, adduction, rotation and circumduction.

The movements can be

symmetrical, identical on each side of the midline of the body, or

asymmetrical, when the arms and/or legs move in different ways.

All movements can be with a small or large range of motion. This affects choreography as well as intensity.

Play with the upper body movements
For a change try choreographing an eight-count series of arm movements independantly of the leg movements. Then put the arm movements together with some (new) leg movements. The result is a very different, challenging combination.

Active muscles

An important element of the choreography is the number of active muscles: How many body parts move at the same time?

In dance fitness normally you concentrate on the larger muscles of the legs, arms and core.

For variety and added difficulty you can engage more muscles:

Head/neck, shoulders, arms, hands, fingers and feet move – at the same time or alternating.

Example:

Walk, turn 1/1 to the right, arms wave, head shakes (1-4). Stay in place 4 (5-8): Hips side to side, heel-raises, arms to the side, curl the fingers, turn the head left and right.

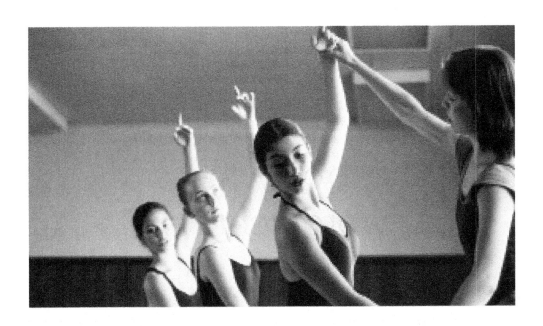

Style

Apart from these seven variations, dance fitness choreography can be changed even further by adding style:

Stylize the movements, so they accentuate and interpret the chosen music and the mood of the music.

If you choose original music in different genres – as opposed to pre-mixed music with an added base rhythm – you experience a certain feeling, which can be transferred to the movements.
The music sets the mood.

The instructor can plan for stylized moves in advance, but with original inspirational music, many new details can evolve spontaneously.

Modern dance, jazz dance, gymnastics and ballet can provide inspiration for dance fitness classes as well as cardio based classes such as aerobics or power dance.

Funk, latin and dance are the three main music genres in group exercise fitness dance; some basic styling suggestions:

"The body says what words cannot."

Martha Graham (1894-1991)

Funk

Syncopated, accentuated movements with lots of hip and core movement with *contraction* of the mid-section of the body. The movements are somewhat heavy and percussive.
The body language can be cool, relaxed, with *attitude*.

Latin

Syncopated small, rather fast movements with the hips, legs and shoulders. The movements are 'light' and suggestive. The body excudes sensual energy and joy for dancing.

Dance

Dance can be *modern*, inspired by modern dance, *retro* with a disco or showdance look – or *powerdance* with intense gymnastic steps, poses and jumps.

Tip: Find themes and steps in dance moveis and soaps such as Glee, Fame, Saturday Night Fever, Flashdance, All that jazz, and music videos by a.o. Michael Jackson.

The dance/exercise style should fit the music; is it happy 80's disco, cool 90's dance or 00's relaxed lounge?

Style is everything
Avoid *"trying too hard"*. If the movements are too forced and sharp, the dance may seem awkward. Style is characterized by control of the body and moves in harmony with the music.

Combinations

In dance fitness choreography you can select and combine the base moves, first step by step and then block by block, for an almost infinite number of combinations:

- Select basic steps.

- **Combine basic steps into an eight-count,** a phrase, a selection of steps corresponding to eight beats of music. Eg. eights steps of 1 beat each, four steps of 2 beats each, two steps of 4 beats each or mixed.

- **Combine four eight-counts to a block,** 4 x 8 beats, of choreography. Blocks are named, A, B, C, D etc. Note, the blocks fit verses as well as choruses.

- **Combine three or more blocks,** normally eight is maximum, for a complete dance fitness choreography.

- Add style or variations to the basic steps.

- **Combine the basic steps with torso and upper body movements.** These can also be stylized.

You may also choreograph intuitively without thinking about eights and blocks. Ask: ***"What moves can the body do?", "What does the music tell you to do?"***

No one method is better than another, however, the above process is highly recommendable in dance fitness as it is easy to approach and it 'gets the job done'...

Blocks in fitness

In group exercise, e.g. a funk or power dance class, the instructor often creates a choreography of **3-4 blocks.**

The 3-4 blocks are normally taught starting first with a right leg lead, then with a left leg lead.
In this way you get a nice balanced workout.
However, it takes time to include both right and left leg work, so there is only time for a limited number of blocks.

Block choreography also requires a certain level of concentration, so you remember the steps and sequence of the blocks.

Tip: Give each block its own identity via a step or a theme; do it for variety and for making each block easier to remember.

Blocks in dance

In dance (fitness) you seldom repeat (mirror) whole blocks of choreography. Rather you make a small choreography for each piece of music, e.g. **8-10 blocks.** Blocks are not combined or repeated with the other leg, but there may be mirrored steps within the block.

When choreographing for fitness dance, you should – for balanced workouts – have a similar number of steps for the right and left leg. Example:
If in block A you have an asymmetrical series with four skips with the right leg and none with the left, later on in block B, C or D, do four skips with the left; either throughout the blocks or in one block.
You do not need to perform identical steps or have a perfect match, as long as there is some balance.

Transitions

Dance fitness classes with flow are characterized by a smooth linking of all steps and blocks of movements.

A transition can be:

- Fluent (invisible)
- Frozen
- Fun
- Fantastic

Fantastic transitions can be jumps and leaps etc. Stop in a pose or continue without stopping.

Fun transitions can be sudden, unexpected and fun (cartoon) figures.

Frozen positions are like still life *'freeze frames'*. Hold for 2-4 beats or more.

Fluent or invisible, smooth transitions are the norm in group exercise.

The goal of transitions:

1) The final choreograpy is harmonious and it flows.

2) During class the choreography is built with flow; the steps flow together, so that nobody misses a beat or stops.

This is achieved by:

- Harmony between music and exercises.

- Logical sequencing.

- Natural travel patterns and direction changes.

- Movements fit together; the end of one move flows into the beginning of the next move.

- Combinations starting with a right foot lead continues into other right foot combinations. The same thing applies for left foot lead combinations.

From right to left

In dance fitness there are two primary methods – apart from steps like ball-change and chassé – for transitioning from a right foot lead sequence to a left foot lead sequence

- Neutral steps
- Lift steps (step lifts)

Neutral steps

Neutral steps bring both legs together and distribute the bodyweight evenly across the feet.
Examples:
Stand, jump, jack, twist, plié or squat.

After a neutral step, you can continue moving in any direction. This means, though, that the instructor has to tell the participants precisely, in short, and in time, which leg to use, which way to go.

Lift steps (step lifts)

You can change the lead leg, e.g. from left to right, with an uneven number of repetitions of a lift step.

For instance a lift step with the rhythm single, single, double – three lifts total – equals one eight-count of choreography; this results in a fluent transition from one lead leg to the other.

A lift step in which the lift, e.g. skip, hamstring curl, kneelift or kick, is repeated is called a *repeater*.

A repeater can have two, three, four, five or seven lifts. Preferably not more than this, as it is hard on the supporting leg knee.

In dance fitness doubles, repeater 2's, are popular in combination with other steps, e.g. step, double knee, jack 2.

Organisation

The choreography can have several different positions during class. Ask **Where? Who? What?**

Where?
The instructor and the exercisers can be in various positions in different places in the room.

With Whom?
One and one, in pairs or in groups, diverse formations or acrobalances.

With What?
You can use *props* or fitness equipment such as benches, balls or ropes.

Normally you do not use props in dance fitness, but they are great for shows and demos and can be used for showing the diversity of fitness. *Note: In showdance – and lady and strip fitness – e.g. chairs and poles are used as props.*

Formation: The way the participants are grouped, e.g. in a triangle or circle formation.
This is an important element of show choreography.

Position: The way the participants are positioned in relation to each other, e.g. within a formation two or more participants can change places with each other.

The organization of the class has a major effect on the dance experience.

Throughout any dance choreography – for group exercise or a show – the positions can change.

In dance fitness the use of various positions within a single class requires, that the instructor has a keen eye and keeps the class moving; keeps the class organized.

In return new, different positions provides new (social) experiences and welcome breaks from the usual (dance) fitness unison group position.

The instructor normally is in front with exercisers positioned around the room. However the instructor and exercisers can move to other places in the room, in small or large groups, facing in different directions.

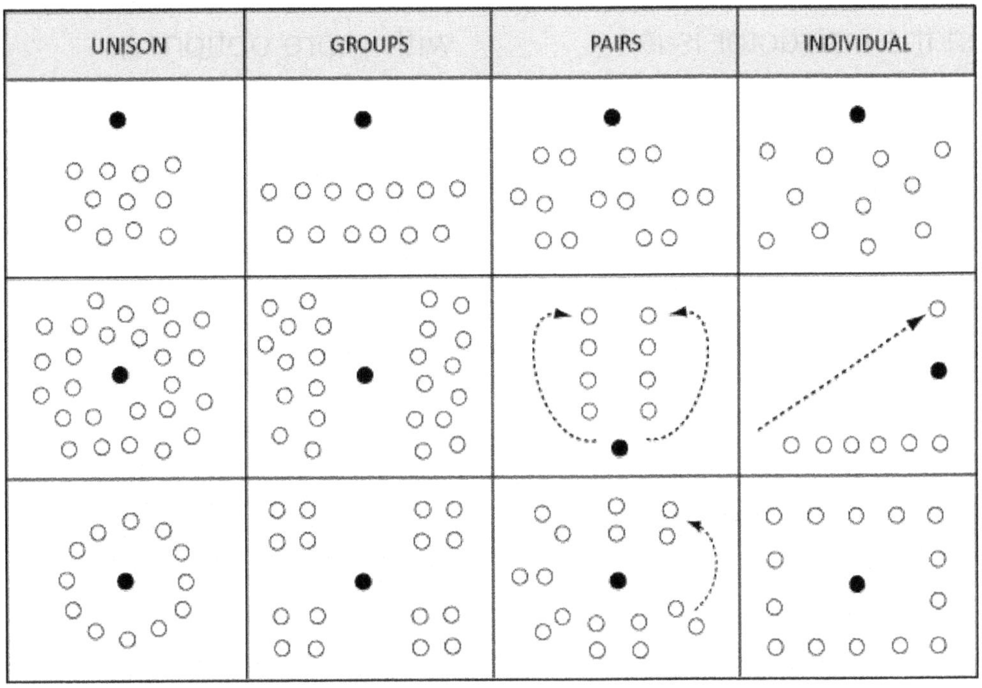

UNISON	GROUPS	PAIRS	INDIVIDUAL

Figure 5.4: Dance fitness formations, and positions. Aagaard.

In unison

In a unison format all the exercisers are doing the same moves at the same time; it is easy for the instructor to get a good view over the class.

In a traditionel unison format with the instructor in front it is possible to teach advanced level choreography even with minimal instruction; it is the preferred format in dance fitness classes.

When the instructor is in the middle of the room or a circle of dancers, the combinations cannot be too complex; when exercisers see each other from different angles, it can be difficult choosing the right lead leg and going in the right direction.

Tip: In a circle: Say *"look to the persons next to you, not those opposite you"*.

One and one

In one and one formats, you are not part of a group or a pair. In dance fitness this means, that everybody works out 'on their own', but everybody are doing the same steps simultaneously.

Another option in one and one training is doing different moves at the same time or the same move at different times:

• Steps and movements with more options, e.g. freestyle.

• Circuit or station training, one and one.

• Follow-the-leader; the instructor or exerciser shows a move, which is then performed by everybody. Example: Run in a diagonal line across the room one at a time.

Groups

In a 'groups' format, the participants are divided into small or large groups, close to each other or in different formations, e.g. rows, lines and circles.

Lines, two or more, are fun and at the same time the instructor still has a good view over the class. Several groups around the room is also an option, but the instructor must be extra attentive to keep everybody moving.

Two groups facing each other:

Option 1: dance with *right and left leg* so the two groups move in opposition.

Option 2: with the side to the front and back wall; dance with *front and back leg,* so the two groups are mirroring each other.

Pairs

Partner work is a great option, which can be very motivating.
You create a sense of community, which may result in better adherence.

In pairs you can work together, help each other, assist, or resist, and even compete to perform better.

Note: Partner work must be introduced in the right way, and gradually, so the participants feel at ease.

Partner – and group – formats allows for inter-actions and even acro balances, which is a natural part of show choreography.
Acro balances can be simple lifts in standing, kneeling, sitting or lying position or they can be advanced sports acro balances.

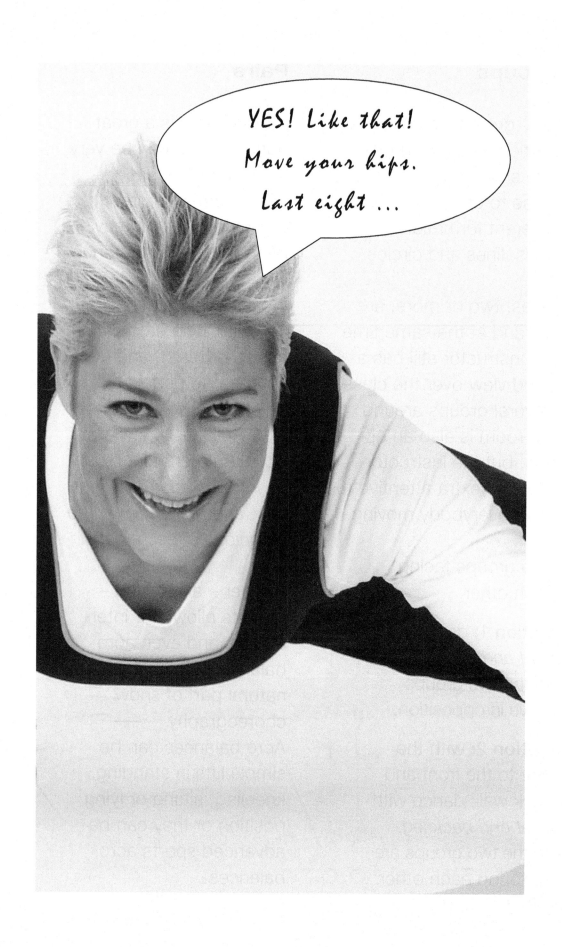

Chapter 6 | **Methodology**

Succesful dance fitness is not just about the moves; actually many of the most popular classes are *not* the ones with the better choreography ...
What motivates and makes participants want to come back is the millieu created by the instructor: A feeling of success and a feeling of belonging.

Fortunately most people join dance fitness classes for fun, because they are motivated to do so and not because they have to, which is often the case in traditional fitness training. Still several people drop out, because they lose motivation; sometimes because they feel lost or unnoticed; feel that the instructor does not notice them ... even if this is not so at all.

Motivation

Everybody needs to feel:

- Competence (success)
- Control (have options)
- Relatedness (belong)

Internal motivation, which make you participate for fun, is fuelled by:

- Learning something
- Improving or accomplishing something
- Feeling, sensing something

Instructors can promote the feeling of happiness and success by being aware of the above and via dynamic enthusiastic teaching methods;
1) keep (eye)contact with all of the exercisers,
2) keep everybody moving
3) communicate (dialogue) in a positive, open way.

Methods

In dance (fitness) the teaching methods and the learning process is essential; how, how much and how fast (do dancers master the moves). The right methodology is essential for a good result; happy dancers.

Some of the primary tasks of the instructor; to 1) create a positive environment, 2) teach in a way, so that dancing seems logical and easy and 3) teach moves at different levels, differentiate.

In order to ensure flow, you should prepare a 'flexible' choreography and pay attention to the reactions of the dancers and then make adjustments as necessary.

Instructors have almost limitless posibilities for motivating and engaging the participants; strategy:

- Preparation, a plan.

- Gradual progression.

- One thing at a time.

- Diverse methods for coaching and delivering the choreography.

- Clear and precise execution and cueing, so that everybody can see, hear and follow.

- Positive introductions of novel steps; 'new', 'fun', 'different': Avoid 'difficult', 'necessary' or *"we have to learn these first ..."*.

The more gradual and easy the progression initially, the faster and easier the learning proces will be onwards.

Progression

Gradual progression is essential; for each dance class and throughout the season, there should be a progression.
Progression meaning, that you start at an easy level and progress onto harder or more difficult variations over time.

How quickly to progress and develop the dances, depends on the skill level of the participants.

Note: If a club or studio has a general description of classes with set levels of difficulty, the instructor must adhere to this.

Dance for fitness classes should have moves, that are **differentiated**; moves should be demoed at 2-3 levels, so exercisers can choose the version, they prefer – or can perform.
In show choreography, there are no options; everyone performs the planned choreography.

In dance **battle,** two groups of dancers 'battle' to show off the series, perform or compete.
Battle requires, that the dancers feel confident, are not uneasy about performing, otherwise the result is frustration!

Examples of progressions

Walk > walk with a bounce > walk with a double hop

Step touch > triple step > triple step with turning

Step tap > step kneelift > step piruette

Walk out and in > stepout-jack > jack > off beat jack

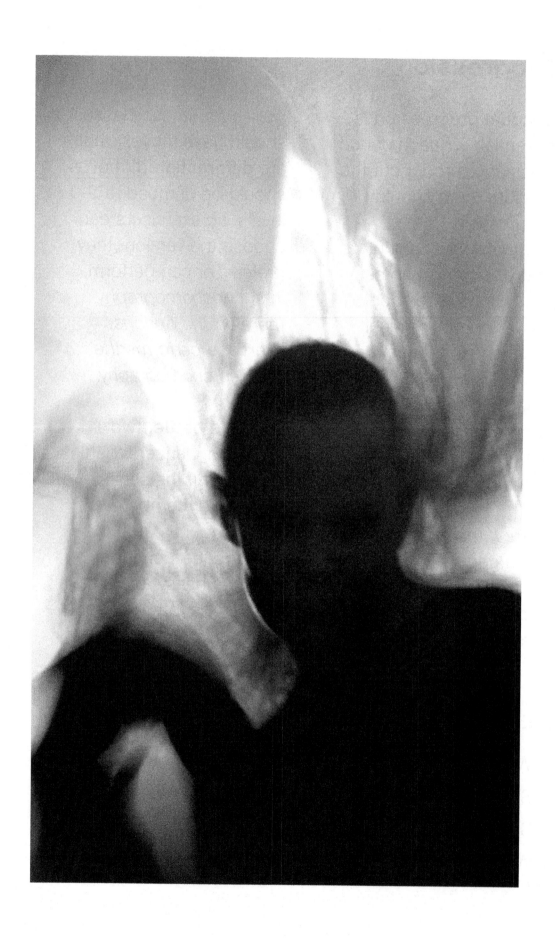

Combination building

During class the dance instructor should teach using the part-to-whole principle;
by teaching one part at a time, the class will progress much faster.

Keywords for smooth combination building:

- **Fluent action** without stops and rest-pauses.

- **Balance between exercises**; an even distrubution of right and left side move-ments – even in asym-metrical blocks.
  This feels motivating and natural.
  Too many repetitions with the same leg can result in fatigue and impatient exercisers.

- **Everybody is active**
  keep everyone moving; differentiate the moves.

- **Logical and ordered composition**. Ideally blocks should be built with the *same number of basic steps with the same rhythm and in the same place as in the final version.*
  Avoid detours and wasting time learning something, that does not belong or belongs somewhere else.

- **Manageable layout**
  It is difficult to learn a lot in a short time; learning is easier in small doses; e.g. parts of 8-16 beats, which are then added.

- **Flexible program**
  There are many ways of teaching dance:
  Choose your method according to the steps, the context and group.
  Change tactics along the way if necessary.

Freestyle

In freestyle you improvise without aiming for an end product.
This is a great way of dancing or working out with room for experiments and surprises.

Moves can be built and linked intuitively using the linear progression principle or combined into short patterns with no combination building. The advantage is, that you do not have to learn or memorize longer sequenses.

Freestyle works best, when the instructor has a large repertoire of moves, so the class does not get boring.

Linear progression

You start with one step or move and change one thing at a time, arm or leg movements, rhythm, direction or travelling.
You do not repeat moves in a pattern or blocks and you do not have an end product.
This way the choreography flows and is easier to master.

Linear progression can be used in warm-ups and in between block building.
If this method is used for most of the class, the instructor must be good at changing only one thing at a time and have a large repertoire of exercises in order to keep coming up with different moves.

Use different teaching methods to make exercisers more proficient and open to new approaches.

Block building

Block building is the pre-ferred method in group exercise.

First you build, teach, one block, to fit 4 x 8 counts of music, then the next block, which is added, and so on.

Example:
First you build block A, then B. The two are then linked. Then the next two blocks, C and D, are built and linked with blocks A and B:

A   built
B   built
A+B   are added
C   built
D   built
C+D   are added
A+B+
C+D   are combined

Normally there are 3-4 blocks in an intermediate level group exercise class.

Verse-chorus choreo-graphy is used in concept classes (and gymnastics); for every song, normally 6-12 songs, you compose a part, block, for verses, A parts, the chorus, B part, and bridge, C part.

The blocks, the final choreography, can be built during a single class or develop over several classes depending on the level of difficulty and skill level of the participants.

Example, music analysis:

A   Verse
B   Chorus
A   Verse
B   Chorus
C   Bridge
A   Verse
B   Chorus
C   Bridge
A   Verse
B   Chorus
B   Chorus

Block building tips

Give each block its own identity; avoid doing mambo, chassé and kneelift in all blocks. Make each block different. This provides variation and makes it a lot easier to distinguish and remember the blocks apart.

Name every block after its special characteristics; this makes it easier to learn and remember each block (Kennedy-Armbruster, Yoke, 2009).

Mirror method and mix and match

In group exercise you learn each block with either the left or right leg as the leading leg, and then move on to the next block. Or you mirror the block, performing each block with first one leg according to the choreography and then mirror it with the other leg.
This is the dominant method at present.
Note: For fluent transitions from right to left leg lead, somewhere in the block, there should be a lift step or neutral step, that changes the lead leg.

Advantage: The muscles get a balanced workout.

Disadvantage: The class, choreography, becomes quite predictable and there is less variation.

After the complete choreography has been learned, it can be performed in its entirety with right and left leg lead alternating. This works well with an uneven number of blocks, usually three; right, left, right leg starts block A, B, C. Then left, right, left leg starts.

Layering

First you build the choreography; blocks of 4 x 8 with easy basic moves.

Then you add a 'layer' on top of one or more of these eights.

The added layer(s) will increase the intensity or level of coordination:

Layers are changes in tempo, rhythm, direction, travelling, planes and joint movement, but without adding more beats of choreography.

Layering is suitable for mixed classes with exercisers at different levels: Each exerciser chooses which layer, level, to follow.

Example:
Skip 4
High Impact skip 4
HI skip, full turn OTS 4

Reverse pyramid principle

Reverse pyramid principle, or reduction, is one of the primary methods.
You start out with many repetitions, which you then gradually reduce to fewer according to this pattern: 8-4-2-1.
This makes it is easy to learn and master even complex combinations.

Example:
Jog 8, easy walk 8.
Jog 4, easy walk 4.
Jog 2, easy walk 2.
Jog 1, easy walk 1.

Pyramid principle

This principle is used in warm-ups. Steps or combinations are repeated more and more times.

Example:
Step touch R/L
Step touch 2 R, 2 L
Step touch 4 R, 4 L

Transitions and links

Pre-composed choreography, with attention to details and transitions is the basis for a great end product, finale, and is of course important.

However, the process, everything leading up to that 'finale', is even more important. So:

Attention has to be on the now; go for fun all the way:

The majority of class is spent building the parts, so it makes a difference, when the class flows smoothly without any rest-pauses or stops: All moves should be built and linked with flow, smooth transitions; this ensures continuity and makes dancing more fun. This is possible, when the instructor instructs with competent cueing.

The Finale
Dance fitness classes can be composed of typical block choreography or **verse-chorus choreography**; verse-chorus choreography can be:

1) 8-10 small independent choreographies, one for each piece of music. After each song, you move on.

2) 1 pre-composed choreography, which is built all the way through class to different pieces of music, unlike e.g. showdance classes, where you use the same song. At the end of class the choreography is performed in its entirety to the original piece of music; the 'finale'.

Plan for fantastic flow and fun fitness dance:

- **Logical**, systematic combination building.

- **Consistent** use of the same names for steps and moves and same way of counting, so participants know, what is coming and when.

- **Precise cueing.** Clear and timely visual and verbal cueing and feedback.

- **Manageable progression:** Change only one thing at a time. arm or leg movement, style or direction etc.

- **Perfectly linked movements.** Position torso, arms or legs in the right position; the end of one move flows into the start of the next move, movements should continue without interruption.

- **Visible transitions.** Transitions should feel 'invisible', but exercisers must be able to notice the moves or changes in time. There will be a stop or break, if the instructor, on a sudden whim, decides to change lead by simple tapping the foot on the floor, which is hard to see from the back of the room.

- **Right and left leg logic.** The right leg starts and continue with right-leg-combinations, while the left leg continues with left-leg-combinations.
  This seems obvious. However, this is not always what happens, unless the dance instructor in advance has planned how to change lead and direction.

Cueing

Cueing is a common term for verbal or visual instruction(s) in group exercise classes.
It is also used as a general expression for teaching and is an important part of teaching dance fitness.

Cueing can be:

- Visual
- Verbal
- Manual

The participants learn faster and better, if the instructor uses both visual and verbal cueing.

Manual instruction, using the hands when giving feedback, is mostly used in strength and flexibility training and for correcting details in dance and is not covered here.

Apart from movement cues the instructor can use peptalk, motivating words, countdowns in unison, clapping, snapping and exaggerated movements.

Note: The posture and body language of the instructor is an important part of visual cueing.

Competent cueing is precise and quickly conveys:

- What (steps and moves)
- How (technique, style and rhythm)
- How many and when (timing)
- Where and where to (position and travelling)

Visual cueing

A major part of communication is visual, non-verbal.
Visual cueing includes movement demonstrations and arm, hand and finger signalling and also your body language ...
In group exercise you use special *cue signs*, used internationally.

There are **movement signs** for some common exercises (page 83), but not all, so be creative. Examples: Kneelift, point to the knee and raise the hand. Hamstring curl, point to the heel and clap your buttocks.

A visual **countdown** is an important cue; when counting down verbally, the instructor holds up the hand and via the number of fingers shows how many repetitions are left; when to change.

Directional cues is an easy and important form of visual cueing: Use the arms and hands to show the direction; left, right, forward, back, up or down.

Visual cueing should be clear and visible.

- Arm(s) high in the air, so everybody can see.

- In countdowns spread your fingers out, so it is clear, if four, three or two repetitions are left.

- Verbal and visual cues must match each other, otherwise the exercisers will be confused and unable to understand.

- The cueing should be open and encourage dialogue and feedback.

Visual preview

A visual preview is when you demonstrate moves in advance; the instructor shows the coming step(s), while the exercisers watch while doing simple steps. In dance fitness for fitness and fatburning, previews should be avoided or limited to max. 1-2 times per class. Otherwise exercisers tend to get bored.
Exception: When cueing complex choreography, you can save time with a visual preview.
Many moves, however, are taught faster and easier without previews.

Previews includes slow motion demonstration: This should be avoided as a general rule, as 1) it makes the steps look more difficult, than they are and 2) the heart rate drops quickly, when the exercisers slow down. Limit or avoid half tempo and slow motion demos.

Tip: During warm-ups it is a good idea to include rehearsal moves for some select steps; this can be done by performing a few repetitions in half tempo or slow motion.

Use body language and visual *and* verbal cueing
Use visual, non-verbal, cueing in stead of too much talk. Give exercisers a chance to enjoy the music.
Do, however, use verbal cues when needed, as dance requires cueing of rhytm and direction changes.
Precise verbal cues make it easier for the exercisers to follow in time and feel successful.
If exercisers are unable to hear or understand the cues in time, they are caught on the wrong foot ...

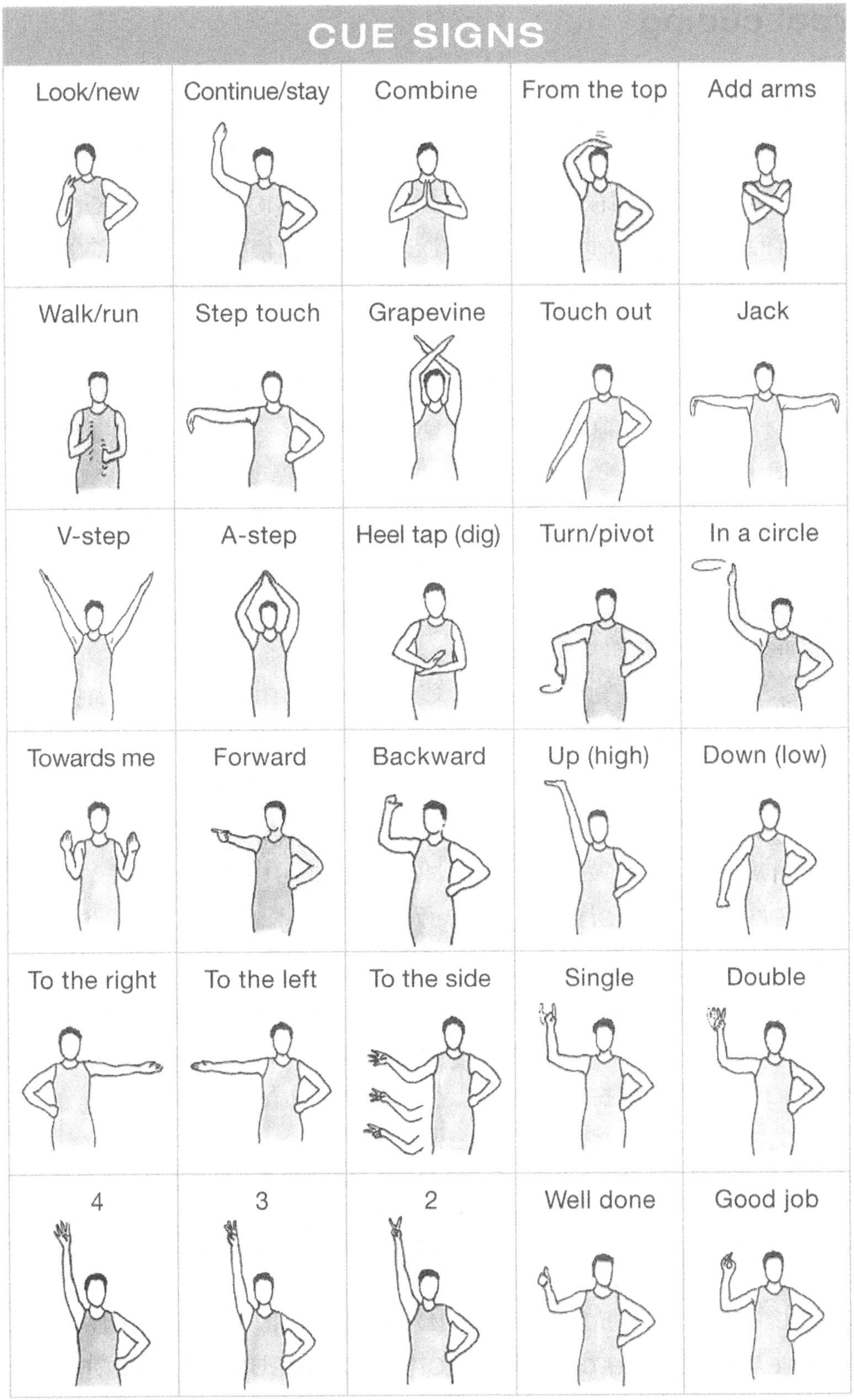

CUE SIGNS

Look/new	Continue/stay	Combine	From the top	Add arms
Walk/run	Step touch	Grapevine	Touch out	Jack
V-step	A-step	Heel tap (dig)	Turn/pivot	In a circle
Towards me	Forward	Backward	Up (high)	Down (low)
To the right	To the left	To the side	Single	Double
4	3	2	Well done	Good job

Figur 6.1: Group exercise cue signs for visual instruction. Aagaard, 2000.

Verbal cueing

Verbal cueing is spoken instructions.
They can be made more interesting and easier to hear by changing the tone of voice, the volume, tempo and accent.
You can keep cues motivating and effective by using different words.

Movement name cueing is sufficient for advanced dancers, but for beginners you must use some **descriptive cueing**; e.g. explain steps and moves. *Note: Explanations, which are understood by one exerciser, may be incomprehensible to another.*

Use images, as it often makes the cues easier to understand.

Examples: "Hunch your back like a *cat*", *"Hold the arms as embracing a ball"*, *"Push the walls out"*.

Instructors should also cue **direction**, which way to turn or move; forward, backward, right, left, diagonally, up or down. And cue lead leg; "right foot starts". If several exercisers are out of time: Use a cue like *"Right foot leads now"*, to get everybody on the beat and using the same lead leg, before moving on.

Countdowns are just that ... you count down.
You do not count up, as exercisers will not know how many reps are left. When the instructor says *"eight", you know that something new is about to happen and that it happens after 8 counts.* Then you cue "four, three, two". Not *"One", instead you cue the next move.*

Exception: In dance you often count up just before changing: *"...5, 6, 7, 8".*

Tip: Use countdowns logically and consistantly: Count down for every repetition of a move.

Examples:

In **running** each footstrike equals a beat. *You do not count continuously, but do cue the exact number.*

In **step touch** count for every step touch; a step touch right and left are two repetitions, not one.

In **grapevine,** grapevine one way is one repetition, returning back is another.

Tip: Draw attention to steps via your voice: count out loud and clear, accent special parts: Stress the number, count, of selected steps;

cueing by numbers

as in counting: *"One-and-**two**-and-three-and-**four**".*

This way the exercisers have no trouble hearing and getting ready to move at the right time. E.g. *"-and-1"* and *"1-and-"* differs and the instructor should cue this.

Use images and guideposts
Directional cues are "forward", "backward", "right", "left", "diagonal", "up" or "down". The instructor can also use things in the room to specify direction, e.g. *"to the door", "towards the clock"* or *"to the stereo".* In this way the exercisers will follow faster.
When turning, especially full turns within one or two beats, where you may lose your sense of direction, it is important with precise directional cueing, like: *"Turn backwards around the left shoulder".*

Verbal preview

Verbal preview is advance information about the movements to come.
If this is done at all, it should be short and precise, because:

Longer verbal cues, previews, are largely a waste of time and information, as most is missed or forgotten.

Example:
If you are starting over, repeating a block already mastered, you should *not* waste time on cueing it in details. It is enough to mention the step or move at the beginning of the part: *"Start over; chassé"*.

The step name should be called to make it clear, if you are starting from the start of the present block or the very first block.

Voice control

The voice is made in the throat, when air from the lungs passes the vocal cords. The sound is turned into speach in the throat and mouth.

The voice can be used in a healthier way and you can avoid getting a sore throat, if you speak with proper breathing and control of the voice.

Using the voice the wrong way, can lead to hoarseness and pain in the neck area. In some cases you risk losing your voice or experience chronic pain.

If you experience hoarseness or pain in the throat, give your voice a rest.
When the pain recides, you can start speaking again in small doses.
If this does not help, you should seek professional help.

Let Your Voice Be Heard

- **Inhale deeply** before speaking.
- **Smile with your voice**; you relax and seem friendlier.
- **Open your mouth well** to get more sound out.
  Your head and mouth act as a loudspeaker
- **Relax the neck and the facial muscles.**
- **Drink sips of water;** moisten your throat, vocal cords.
- **Minimize the use of verbal cueing** and use more
  visual cueing to save your voice.
- **Limit continuous talk and counting**; it is unnecessary.
- **Limit superfluous talk, words;** do not waste your voice.
- **Save your voice** by giving short cues.
- **Draw attention by claps, snaps,** whistles a.o.
- **Use body language,** exaggerate moves; easier to see.
- **Use visual cueing** as often as possible.
- **Play with your voice.** Speak slow, fast, low, high.
- **Inhale deeply and give a shout from time to time.**
- **Avoid lowering your voice unnaturally,** use normal pitch.
- **Use the music smartly,** talk during instrumental parts.
- **Avoid turning the volume up too loud;** keep the
  volume at a sensible level, so your voice is heard.
- **Turn the music down during important cues.**
- **Use less treble,** so your voice is heard more easily.
- **Use a microphone whenever possible** and use it
  wisely. Never shout or whistle into the microphone!

Feedback

Feedback, follow-up and performance cues, helps exercisers improve their movements aesthetically and functionally.
Feedback – general or individual – should be given in a positive and constructive way.

If several exercisers in a group make the same mistake, give general feedback.
If one participant makes a mistake, give individual feedback. However the instructor may opt for general feedback in order not to expose a person. But if he or she does not respond, some sort of direct individual feedback is necessary.

Note: Rebukes and negative criticism will almost always result in a negative reception, attitude, and impair learning.

Feedback should be short and precise, a couple of points at the most, if possible with images, which are easily understood by the exerciser.

Feedback can be given as a 'sandwich':
Positive, neutral and positive comments.
1. Start with the positive, e.g. recognition of an exercise well done; this is a smart way of ensuring positive reception of the following information.
2. Give a neutral tip, e.g. what limits optimal performance – avoid negatives.
3. Finish with a positive tip on how to improve, e.g. better alternatives.

Note: Use the mirror, a valuable feedback tool: It shows you/exercisers immediately, if the move looks o.k. compared to the desired execution.

Corrections

Typical corrections should be limited in dance fitness: The primary goal of dance fitness is fun; feeling successful leads to continued motivation.

As a dedicated trainer of course you also want the participants to improve on their execution, so the movements look better and are safer.
Poor performance can be critical e.g. for the knees and lower back.

Faulty exercise execution must not go unnoticed, but should be eliminated via positive feedback.

Do not think of faults as faults, but rather moves, which have not been mastered yet. So do not criticize, but provide cues for better training effect.

Practice makes perfect.

Beginners, who have not learned the steps, often make many mistakes when dancing.
Still, the instructor should give maximum 2-3 tips, corrections per class; those regarding faults, which are critical; which could lead to injury.

There are two reasons for scarce corrections:

- **It is difficult to learn many new things all at once;** if you correct several technique mistakes at a time, most of these cues will not be remembered and the faults remain.

- **It results in a negative experience, when new exercisers are corrected again and again** instead of being able to have fun and enjoy the dancing.

Mirroring

Motivating communication involves eye contact. As a general rule dance fitness instructors should face their participants

Unfortunately it is quite common for dance and group exercise instructors to have their back to the exercisers.
Even with mirrors, this is bad for communication:

Contact and motivation is very limited. Even if the instructor thinks it is easy to see everyone, some are right behind and see only the back of her/him.

Participacts are 'farther away'; the image of the participants has to travel twice the distance, when it has to pass the mirror to reach the eyes of the instructor. This makes it difficult to spot details and eye contact is limited.

The voice is harder to hear. The sound waves are directed to the mirror instead of towards the participants. Hence it is necessary for the instructor to shout (louder) to be heard.
Even when using a microphone it is helpful, when exercisers can see the mouth of the instructor.

Professional instructors motivate participants by facing them as much as possible: During the entire warm-up, cool-down and stretching and sections of – or most of – the dancing.

Beginners: It is easy to teach an entire class for beginners facing them.

Advanced dancers: They know you and dancing, so when doing multiple turns and intricate steps, often it is better to move with them.

Mirroring tips

When the instructor faces the exercisers, all moves should be mirrored – and verbal as well as visual cueing should take this into account.

Note: When participants should walk with the right leg, the instructor cues "Walk with the right leg", but marches with the left.

It is not difficult to teach as a mirror image and most steps are easily learned by all exercisers.

Tip: Until confident the instructor does not have to say too much about left and right, just point in the right direction.

"What if participants have to walk forward (in relation to the instructor)?"

There are three methods for different situations:

Complete mirroring

The instructor informs participants, that they should see the instructor as a mirror; when he/she walks forward, they walk forward towards him/her. Disadvantage: In smaller rooms the instructor and front dancers, will walk past each other and have their backs to each other.

Partial mirroring

In certain parts of class the instructor can inform the participants *"Now I am (moving) with you"*. He/she turns and walks with (or in front of) the participants.

Stationary mirroring

For big travelling patterns, e.g. chassé forward, the instructor can perform the moves with a small range of motion or in place and verbally cue participants to move forward.

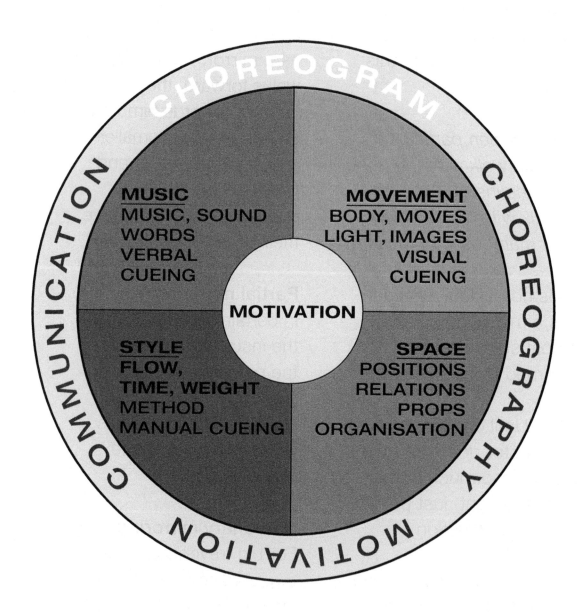

Chapter 7 | **Choreogram**

DANCE FITNESS has presented the basics for composing dance fitness choreography and teaching fun, motivating, effective and healthy dance fitness classes.
The aim is to provide dance fitness instructors with more information, so they can apply new ideas to the areas, where they would like to develop ... as an exercise leader and organizer, teacher or dancer.

The model on the opposite side, *Choreogram* (Aagaard, 2011), sums up, what the dancing experience is about: **Choreography, communication and motivation.**

At the same time it gives a fast overview of the means in composition and learning; music, movements, style and space – along with methodology and cueing.

The book covers several areas, but instructors should not change everything all at once. This seldom works well ...
Take one step at a time: Do not change everything, too much, in your next class. Example: Going from moving with the exercisers to facing them all way through. Even if this is better (for beginners), exercisers need time to adapt.
Tip: In every class change, add or improve just one thing: A technique, a step, a sign or a word. This makes teaching easier and more fun for you *and* for the participants.

For more inspiration the last part of the book, from page 99, has ideas for steps, upper body moves and stretches.

Enjoy!

Litterature

Books | Recommended reading

Alter; MJ (1997), *Sports Stretch, 2nd Edition*, Human Kinetics.

Kennedy-Armbruster, Yoke (2009). Methods of Group Exercise Instruction. Human Kinetics.

Kjoebek, Tybjerg-Pedersen, Tybjerg-Pedersen (1997). *Gymnastik og Dans*. Gyldendahl.

Aagaard, M (2008), *Aerobic - funktionel holdtraening i teori og praksis*. Aagaard.

Aagaard, M (2010), *Fitness og styrketraening*. Aagaard.

Winther, Engel, Noergaard (2001), *Fodfaeste og himmelkys*. Hovedland|Institut for Idraet, Koebenhavns Universitet.

Homepages

us.batuka.com
www.bokwafitness.com
www.breakdance.com
www.dancemagazine.com
www.dynamixmusic.com
www.marinaaagaardblog.com
www.mtv.dk
www.musclemixesmusic.com
www.physicaltunes.com
www.powermusic.com
www.thegroovemethod.com
www.youtube.com
www.zumbafitness.com

Glossary

Abduction	Away from the midline of the body.
Adduction	Towards the midline of the body.
Advanced	Higher level, skilled dancers.
Aerobics	Cardio work (cardiovascular exercise).
Air jack	Explosive jumping jack.
Arabesque	In ballet: On one straight leg, other leg extended back in 90 degree angle.
Attitude	With style. In ballet: Standing on one straight leg, other leg is lifted and bent.
Basic	Base, foundation, starting point.
Battle	Two groups show or 'fight' each other, show off the best performance.
Beat	Music rhythm.
Block	Part of choreography, 4x8 beats.
Bounce	Easy jogging move.
BPM	Beats per minute. Music tempo.
Break	Pause. Stop.
Breakdown	Teach choreography, part-to-whole.
Bridge	Connecting part, e.g. in music.
Cardio-	Concerning the heart.
Cardio-phase	The cardiovascular training part.
Chorus	Composition, refrain, group of people.
Circuit	Training format; a circuit with stations.
Circumduction	Circular movement.
Composition	Choreography, class design.
Core training	Training the core muscles.
Contraction	Contracting, e.g. the abs as in funk.
Cooldown	Bring the heart rate to resting level.
Countdown	Counting down (from eight or four).

Cueing	Instruction, cue words.
Curve	Non-linear. Bending the spine.
Demi-plié	Wide squat, half (grand) plié. Heels down.
Double	Two repetitions in a row, 'two-repeater'.
Eight (count)	Phrase of choreography of 1x8 beats.
Effort	Exertion. Laban: Base quality.
Exercise	To train, workout, fitness move.
Extension	Extending a joint.
Flex	Bending a joint. Contract a muscle.
Flexion	Bending (a joint).
Floorwork	Exercises on the floor, calisthenics.
Formation	Organized in a pattern, e.g. a circle.
Freestyle	Free as opposed to planned, fixed.
Go	Start, go ahead, get moving, move.
Grand plié	Deep wide squat (sumo squat).
Grapevine	Basic move, step out-cross behind-out-together.
HI	High impact.
High	As opposed to low (intensity, impact).
High impact	(Aerobics with) running and jumping.
Hyperextension	Extend beyond normal (neutral).
Intermediate	Middle level, some experience.
Isolations	Isolated, with few muscles involved.
Jack	Jumping jack, jump variation.
Jam	Improvise. Music, dance, free style.
Jump	Propulsion, airborne, both feet.
Kick	Straight leg lift (high).
Complimentary	Same side arm and leg move.
Choreography	Dance, dance notation (greek word).
Lead (leg)	Starting (leg); leg starting the series.
Leap	Propulsion, airborne, one foot take-off.
LI	Low impact.

Low	As opposed to high (intensity, impact).
Lunge	Stepping out.
MI	Moderate impact.
Mixed impact	Combination of low and high impact.
Move	Movement, to change position.
NIA	Neuro-Integrative Action, method.
Opposition	Arm and opposite leg move (opposition). In dance; when right leg moves forward, pull left shoulder back.
Passé	Position in which one leg touches the knee of the opposite leg (ballet).
Pattern	Movement series or 'route' on floor.
Peak	Top. The most intensive part of class.
Pirouette	Turning on the ball of one foot.
Pivot	Turn on one or two feet, e.g. walk turn.
Plié	Squat, wide stance (sumo squat).
Point	Extend. Point foot; plantar flexion of foot, flex foot; dorsal flexion.
Position	The place of a person in a formation.
Press	Push.
Push	Press.
Push up	Exercise with elbow extension.
Q-signs	Cueing system, hand/arm signals.
Repeater	Move repeating a non-weightbearing phase, e.g. repeater tap or lift.
Relax	Release, loosen up, let go.
Release	Relax, let go. Dance technique.
Relevé	Lift up on to the toes, e.g. in ballet.
ROM	Range of motion. Amplitude.
Rotation	Turning. Neck/spine: Right and left. Arms and legs: In and out.
Single	One repetition.

Skate	Step (hop) move, armswing opposite.
Skip	Low kick, knee flexion to extension.
Slide	Glide, step. 'Glissade' in ballet.
Solo	In music and dance accented or performed by one person.
Spotting	Fix your gaze on a fixed point during turn(s), e.g. turn the head, eyes, fast to find that point again to stabilize.
Squat	Bending the legs.
Starjump	High jump, arms and legs out.
Step	Leg movement (or equipment, fitness).
Step touch	Popular dance fitness dance step. Step to the side, tap/together.
Stretching	Relaxing the muscles, flexibility.
Syncopation	Off the base rhythm.
T-balance	Balance, torso and free leg horizontal.
Tap	Touch, change.
Team teach	Two or more instructors teaching.
Theme	Recurring chord or series.
Tempo	Speed of music or movement.
Tendue	Leg is moved forward, out, back with the tip of the toes in the floor (ballet).
Touch	Tap. Physical interaction.
Transition	Move(s) linking one move with another.
Tuck jump	High jump, pull the knees up.
Turn	Rotate body to face new direction.
Turnout	External rotation of the femur (leg).

Appendix | **Dance steps**

This section presents an overview of the most popular group exercise and **dance fitness steps**.

The steps are used in latin based dancing, including ZumbaFitness, Batuku, Bokwa, funk and jazz, power dance, aerobics including combat style classes and disco dance.

The steps can be stylized with torso-, arm- and hip-movement according to the music/dance style.

On the first two pages there is a list of common abbreviations used in dance fitness notation and in this list of steps.

The list is alphabetical with a few of exceptions. In order to keep certain steps together, others have been moved one or two places up or down. Have an extra look, if you miss a step.

Note: Under 'note' there are notes telling, if the step is a 1, 2, 4 beat move. This is a general guideline relating to the number of beats, duration, of the base move. There are many more options.

Principles

The number after a basic step or exercise refers to the number of repetition. E.g. walk 4.

A number in parenthesis denotes the number of beats or rhythm (1,2,3,4), (1-4), (1-and-2, 3,4). A number in 'citation' refers to the exact beat number, e.g. step on beat number '8'.

Jog, run and hop equals 1 beat each:
8 jogs = 8 beats.
Step touch = 2 beats.
4 step touch = 8 beats.
Grapevine = 4 beats.
2 grapevine = 8 beats.

Note: Step touch and grapevine going out, one way, is one repetition. Returning is another, new, repetition; in advanced choreography often there is only one repetition of each step or base move.

Abbreviations

L	Left
R	Right
B	Both
U	Up
D	Down
I	In
O	Out
F	Forward
B	Backward
D	Diagonal(ly)
f	Front/in front of; e.g. move leg f
b	Back/behind; e.g. move leg b
o	Out; e.g. move the leg out
X	On the spot, OTS
x	Cross (past)
GV	Grapevine
ST	Step touch
STS	Side to side
Do.	Ditto, the same
Eg	Example given
ROM	Range of motion, amplitude

Music abbreviations

I   Intro
A   Verse (A-part)
B   Chorus (B-part)
C   Interlude (C-part)
O   Outro

T   Theme, main part

i   Instrumental
v   Vocal
s   Solo

d   Drums
f   Flute
g   Guitar
o   Organ
p   Piano
sx   Sax
sy   Synthesizer
t   Trumpet

Db   Double
Tp   Tempo

In dance fitness you analyze and write down the music structure in relation to the phrases, verse lines, in group exercise choreography. This means, that you count and note 'eights', phrases of eight beats of music, which fit the lines of the verses and choruses. Example:
If it says 2 x 8, it corresponds to 4 x 4 beats of music.

A-STEP

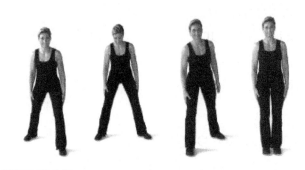

ABDUCTION

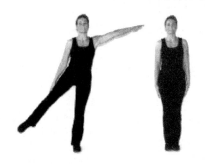

AIR JACK

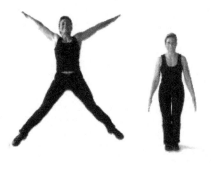

BATMAN

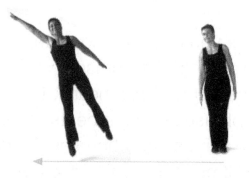

TECHNIQUE	NOTE	VARIATION
A-step. As a V-step mirror image. Feet step back (1), back (2), out wide. Feet step forward (3), forward (4) to closed position. Walk variation.	Four beats. Can also be done as a Step A: Double step touch, diagonally forward, diagonally backward in an A-pattern. Return in the same path.	Tempo Rhythm Direction Joint movement Amplitude, ROM Arm/upper body movements Impact Style
Hip abduction. Lift the leg straight out in frontal plane (1). Range of motion, without moving the pelvis and spine, is approx. 45 degr. Legs together (2). With or without jump.	Two beats. **Side leap and swing** Jump to the side, abduct the leg, land in balance (1), swing the leg in front of support leg (2), leg out (3), legs together (4).	Tempo Rhythm Direction Joint movement Amplitude, ROM Arm/upper body movements Impact Style
A powerful jump into the air with arms and legs out (1). Land with the feet together (2). Can be changed: bent legs, upper body in different positions and various landings.	Two beats. Intermediate to advanced level. Super high impact. Also called **star jump**.	Tempo Rhythm Direction Joint movement Amplitude, ROM Arm/upper body movements Style
Jump with hip abduction (1). Land, legs together (2). On the spot or travelling (to the side). Jump variation.	Two beats. Intermediate level. High impact step. *Note: Jump high and land straight down. Be careful with lateral travelling; watch the knees.*	Tempo Rhythm Direction, Travelling Joint movement Amplitude, ROM Arm/upper body movements Impact Style

BOW AND ARROW

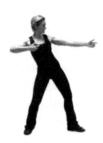

BOX STEP

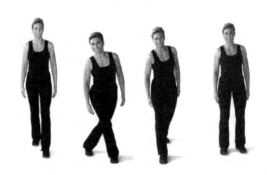

BUTTERFLY

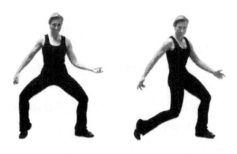

CABBAGE PATCH

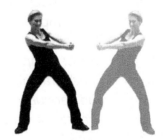

TECHNIQUE	NOTE	VARIATION
Feet wide, rib cage isolation, 'bow and arrow'. Shift torso and shoulder to one side, pull the arm, elbow, out to the same side. Opposite arm straight and in horizontal plane as if holding a bow.	One to two beats. Upper body movement. Alternating, side to side on 1-and- 2-and-.	Tempo Amplitude, ROM Leg position Style
First foot walk forward (1), second foot crosses over (2), first foot steps back, out (3), and second foot steps back (4). Walk variation.	Four beats. Also called **jazz square.**	Tempo Rhythm Direction Joint movement Amplitude, ROM Arm/upper body movements Impact
Feet wide. Rotate legs in (1) and out (2). Heel on the working leg is lifted, so you only touch the ball lightly; it is easier to pivot on the ball of the foot.	Two beats. One or both legs rotate in and out, hip rotation. Working leg foot pivots lightly on the ball of the foot.	Tempo Rhythm, e.g.: R 3, hold/change, L 3, hold/change. R/L/both 2. Arm/upper body movements Style
Feet wide. Circular movements with the upper body; push the chest out and circle the arms opposite in horizontal plane; as if stirring in a large pot.	One to two beats. 'Stirring a pot full of cabbage'. Hands are out and together as if holding a big spoon in a pot.	Tempo Rhythm Style; the base move is a funk move.

CALYPSO BASIC
(ZumbaFitness©)

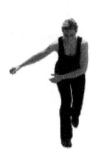

CHA-CHA

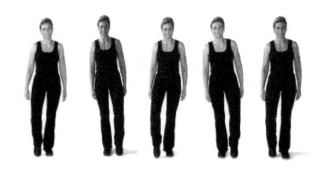

CHA-CHA-CHA

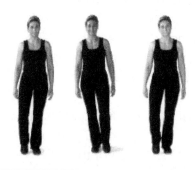

CHASSÉ

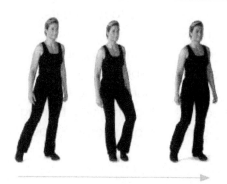

TECHNIQUE	NOTE	VARIATION
Standing. Feet hip-width apart. Lunge forward with one leg, push back to return. The torso leans forward into the movement. Repeat with the opposite leg.	One to two beats. Can be performed in low impact, 'walking' or with a hop during the change from one leg to the other.	Tempo Rhythm Arm/upper body movements Style
Combination of two steps (a tempo), two faster steps, and one step (a tempo). Rhythm 1, 2, 3-and-, 4. Walk variation.	Four beats. Low and moderate impact step.	Tempo Rhythm Direction Travelling Joint movement Amplitude Arm/upper body movements Style
Three little fast steps with the rhythm '1-and-2'. With slightly bent legs and hip movement. Walk variation.	Two beats. Can be used for changing lead leg: An uneven number change legs, an even number keep the same lead leg.	Tempo Rhythm Direction Travelling Joint movement Amplitude Arm/upper body movements Style
Cha-cha-cha with travelling forward, diagonally, backward or to the side. Rhythm: '1-and-2', '3-and-4, etc. Walk variation.	Two beats. Nice for travelling (stay on your toes). Watch the knees during lateral moves. You can do several chassé's to the side: **Boxers shuffle.**	1. Chassé 1-and-2 right, touch L foot behind, walk R foot. 2. Chassé 1-and-2 right, walk/turn 1/1 turn (3, 4). 3. Combo: 1-and-2-and-3-and-4-and + jazz square (5-8).

DANCE FITNESS STEPS

CHARLESTON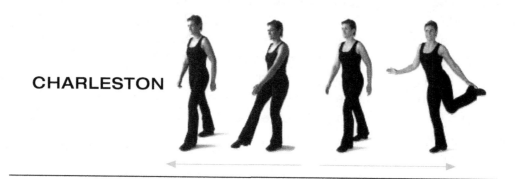

CIRCLES AND TURNS 1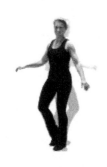

CIRCLES AND TURNS 2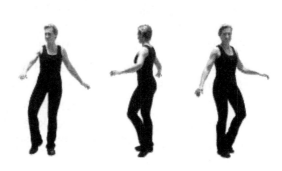

CIRCLES AND TURNS 3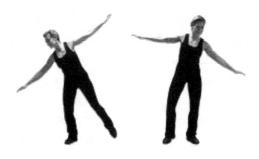

TECHNIQUE	NOTE	VARIATION
Skip, walk, front/back. Variations e.g.: Alternating or doubles. Leg to the side; thigh rotates in, lower leg rotates out, hand to foot. Or; thigh rotates out, lower leg rotates in, hand to foot.	Two or four beats. Four beats: R walk, L skip (variation), L walk, R tap back. Or: Heel kick back/up (1), down/tap (2), back/up (3), down/tap (4).	Tempo Rhythm Direction Joint movement Amplitude Arm/upper body movements Impact Style
Walk on the spot. Turn at the same time, right or left, forward or backward. Variation: First one way, then the other way.	One to eight beats. Nice for balance and spacial awareness, but avoid too many too soon for beginners as they tend to get dizzy.	Tempo Direction; turn: 1/4, 1/2, 3/4,1/2, 1/1, 2/1, 3/1 or more. Arm/upper body movements Style
Walk. At the same time turn and travel; forward, backward, to the side or diagonally.	One to eight beats. Stay on the balls of your feet. Several beats, e.g. turn one way and then the other way. Right or left, forward or backward.	Tempo Direction; turn 1/4, 1/2, 3/4,1/2, 1/1, 2/1, 3/1 or more. Combo: Walk with legs bent and turn 1/1 to the side (1, 2), stand, 'wave', roll up (3, 4).
Walk in 'flexible', curvy patterns, while turning; circles and freestyle. Or linear patterns forward, backward, to the side or triangles and squares with turns.	One to eight beats. Several beats, e.g. turn one way and then the other way. Right or left, forward or backward.	Grapevine with turn: Out, cross behind, out, turn ½ (1/1), together. Out (1), x b, stand (2), turn ½ back (3), feet together (4). GV (1-3), turn 1/4 (4), walk forward 4 (5-8).

DANCE FITNESS STEPS

DESTROZA
(ZumbaFitness©)
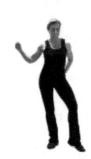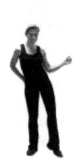

EASY WALK
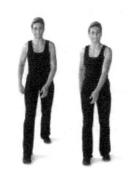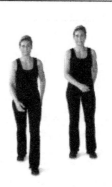

EXTENSION
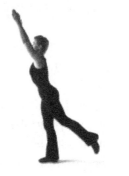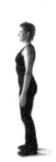

FOOT (LEAD) CHANGE
("AND CHANGE")
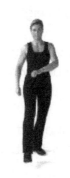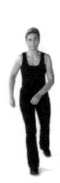

TECHNIQUE	NOTE	VARIATION
Feet wide. One foot stomps in the floor, while hips move side to side. 1-and, 2-and. Arms swing along behind the body as if your are wiping yourself with a towel.	One and a half beat. Intense latin step, stomp hard in the floor, 'destroy'. Watch the knees. Limit the number and intensity of stomps.	Tempo Direction; you can do a 1/4, 1/2 or 1/1 turn, while stomping.
Walk one foot forward (1), step forward to it with the opposite foot (2), walk back with the first foot (3) and walk back with the second foot (4). Walk variation.	Four beats. As a V-step, but with the feet closer to each other, normal stance.	Tempo Rhythm Direction Travelling Joint movement Amplitude, ROM Arm/upper body movements Style
The leg is lifted straight back into hip extension: Extend leg back (1). Bring the leg back to the other, supporting, leg (2).	Two beats. The leg can only move approx. 10-15 degr. back, then movement occurs in the pelvis and spine. Contract the core to stabilize the back.	Tempo Rhythm Direction Travelling Joint movement Arm/upper body movements Impact Style
One foot walks in place, forward or any other direction (-and-), the opposite foot taps lightly in place (1) in order to shift the weight, change lead. Walk variation.	One and a half beat. Requires clear and precise counting and instruction, so the participants notices the change. Part of the step *'kick-ball-change'* (1-and-2).	Tempo Direction Joint movement Amplitude, ROM Arm/upper body movements Impact Style. Use different music. Lift hip with tap.

GALLOP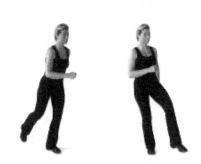

GRAPEVINE (1)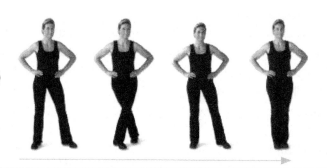

GRAPEVINE (2)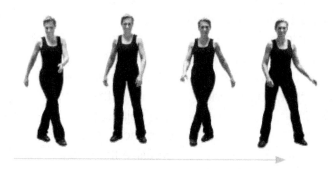

GRAPEVINE (3)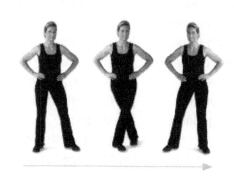

TECHNIQUE	NOTE	VARIATION
One foot in front of the other, 'walk stance', feet move with rhythm; 1-and, 2-and, 3-and, 4-and. As a 'gallop'; rhythm is accentuated by the front foot.	One and a half beat. Walk variation. During forward travelling; front foot moves forward and the back foot closes.	Tempo, Rhythm Direction, Travelling Joint movement Amplitude, ROM Arm/upper body movements Impact Style
First foot out (1), cross second foot behind (2), first foot out (3), close; tap second foot by the first foot (4). Tap can be replaced by a lift step e.g. kneelift. Or a walk step to continue in the same direction.	Four beats. Walk variation. Cross in front or behind. Numerous variations, e.g.: R out (1, 2), L cross behing R (-and-), R out (3), L together (4).	Tempo, Rhythm Direction Travelling Head, arm, body movements, e.g. legs half tempo, arms a tempo. Impact Style
First foot out (1), cross second behind (and), first foot out, continue (2), second foot cross in front (and), first foot out (3), second cross behind (and), first foot out (4). Stop or: Tap second foot (and).	Four beats, eight steps; double tempo step. Move the hips with the movement. From end position, GV return or new steps: e.g. paddle turn 1/1. Photos show last four steps "-and-3-and-4".	**Crosswalk** side (jazzy): Start: Cross right foot in front of left (1), left out (2), cross right in front (3), etc. to the left. E.g. on 4 (two cross over) or 8 (four cross overs), then kick left out ("8"). Return.
Three counts out and return e.g.: Right foot right (1), left foot cross behind (2), right foot right (3), return: left foot out (left) (4), right cross behind (5), left foot left (6). You can add walk 2 (7, 8).	Six (eight) beats. In half tempo, a tempo or double tempo. E.g. two GV, out and back, with turn; diamond shape: GV 3 DR, GV 3 DL, walk 2, turn ½. Repeat, return.	Four beats (funky): Right foot out (1), left cross behind (and), right foot out (2),return: left foot out (left) (and), right foot cross behind (3), left foot out (and), right foot in floor to wide stance (4).

DANCE FITNESS STEPS

HAMSTRING CURL
(SLOW JOG, LEG CURL)

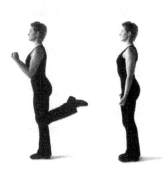

HAMSTRING CURL
(STEP CURL)
(HOP SCOTCH)

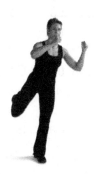

HEELDIG

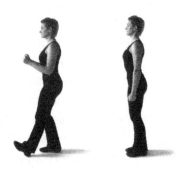

HEELHOP
(HEEL SHUFFLE)

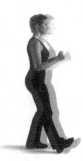

TECHNIQUE	NOTE	VARIATION
Hamstring curl; as a sort of half tempo, low impact jog; pull the heel to the buttocks (1). Feet together (2).	Two beats. Heel to the buttocks on the count of "1". Point foot in top position for 'elegance'. If you flex foot, do so with control; 'funky'.	Tempo Rhythm Direction Travelling Amplitude Arm/torso movements Style
Step or hop out to wide stance (1) as in step curl, hopscotch. Hamstring curl, pull the heel up to the buttocks (2).	Two beats. Heel to the buttocks at the count of "2". Low impact or high impact.	Tempo Rhythm Direction Travelling Amplitude Arm/torso movements Style
Heeldig – or heeltap or heel touch. A tap, dig; heel to the floor (1) and feet together (2).	Two beats. Stylize with arm and torso movements. Slow, heavy, with bent legs. Or light and fast.	Tempo Rhythm Direction, Travelling Joint movement Amplitude Arm/torso movements Impact Style
Heeldig but without bringing feet together. A tap, dig; heel to the floor (1). Hop and repeat with the other foot. Alternating. Or do variations with e.g. repeaters.	One beat. Stylize with arm and torso movements and legs at different angles.	Funky: Double tempo, start by lifting the knee (-and-) and put the right heel (1) and left heel to the floor (-and-2) and right heel to the floor 2 (3,4). Or kick the leg to the side twice (3,4).

HEELJACK

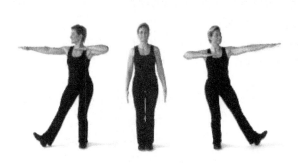

HOP (1)

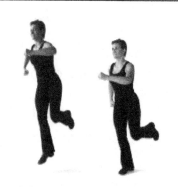

HOP (2)

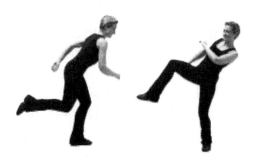

HOPSCOTCH

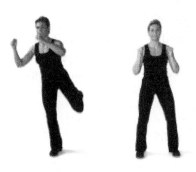

TECHNIQUE	NOTE	VARIATION
As a jumping jack, but heeldig with one foot. From legs together jump legs out, land with one leg bent other leg straight with the heel in the floor (1). Jump legs together (2).	Two beats. As a jumping jack with legs together or legs crossing. Or: One beat: Alternating without closing the legs. Contract the pelvic floor. High impact.	Tempo. Rhythm, Direction Travelling (backwards) Arm/upper body movements Style

Alternating right, left or repeaters. |
| Leap from one foot (1), hop and land on the same foot (2).

Low or high hopping height.

Hop forward, to the side or backward. | Two beats.

In (dance) fitness avoid hopping more than 2-8 times on the same leg, as it is hard on the foot and knee. High impact step. | Tempo. Rhythm, Direction Travelling Arm/upper body movements Style |
| Funky hop: First leg hop forward, kick second leg back (1), stay on first leg, hop turn ½ and kick, frontkick with second leg (2). | Two to four beats.

Hop and kick front to back or side to side. | Hop on first leg, lean forward, kick second leg back (1), hop back, return, and land on the second leg and frontkick first leg (2). |
| Hop or combination of hop and jump. Hop and bend the free leg behind the working leg, hamstring curl (1) and jump out, feet wide (2). | Two beats.

High impact move. | Tempo Rhythm Direction, Travelling Joint movement Amplitude, ROM Arm/upper body movements Impact Style |

DANCE FITNESS STEPS

HUSTLE

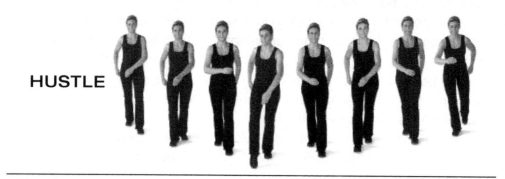

JAZZ STEP

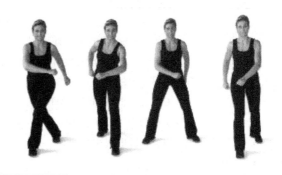

JAZZ TURN

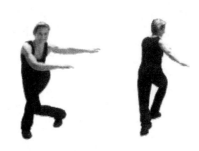

JIG

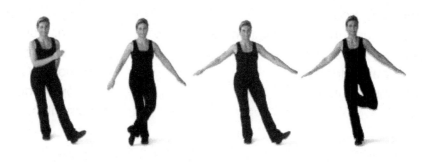

TECHNIQUE	NOTE	VARIATION
Walk three steps forward (1-3), right, left, right. Tap left foot (4). Walk three steps backward (1-3), left, right, left, tap right foot (4). Walk variation.	Four beats. Eight beats forward and back. This step is a low impact step, but impact-variations are possible.	Tempo Direction Joint movement Amplitude, ROM Arm/upper body movements Impact Style
First foot crosses in front (1), second foot steps back (2), first foot back (3), second foot forward (4). Or: First foot forward, second foot crosses in front, first foot back/out, second foot back.	Four beats. Low impact step; jazz step, jazz square, jazzcircle or box step. Perform half tempo with more upper body movement or in double tempo.	1. Half tempo, e.g. two stomps per step. 2. Double tempo, two jazz steps: 1-and-2-and, 3-and-4-and. 3. High impact: Jump up and kick out, land (-and-1), cross over (2), walk back (3,4).
First foot crosses in front (1), second foot back/out and the body starts turning (2), first foot walks to the back wall (3), second foot (body) turns to face front again (4).	Four beats. Low impact step. As a jazz step with a turn. Perform with legs bent and bouncy movements.	Tempo, Rhythm, Direction Joint movement Amplitude Arm/torso movements e.g. when leg crosses over, pull the arms out to the opposite side (horizontal).
Leg to the side, straight leg, heel to the floor (1), bend the leg, toe to the floor in front of other leg (2), heeldig to the side (3), bend the leg, hamstring curl, jump and change legs (4). Repeat other leg.	Four beats. Jig, or gigue, is the name of a lively dance. Perform the steps in a bouncy style, in moderate or high impact.	Tempo Rhythm Direction Travelling Joint movement Amplitude, ROM Arm/upper body movements Style

JACK (1)

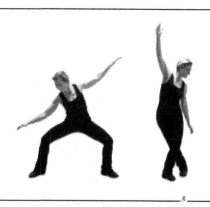

JACK (2)

JACK (3)

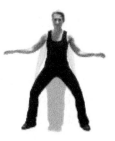

JACK (4)

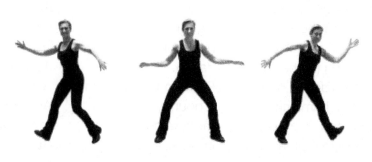

TECHNIQUE	NOTE	VARIATION
Jump out to wide stance (1), jump in, feet together (2). In a narrow, less than shoulder-width, jack, feet point forward. In a wide jack, beyond shoulder-width, feet point slightly outward.	Two beats. Contract the pelvic muscles. Keep knees and feet aligned. Base step. High impact. Can travel, also to the side and forward, but watch the knees.	Tempo, Rhythm, Direction, Travelling (typically backwards) Joint movement Amplitude, ROM Arm/upper body movement Impact Style
Jump out to wide stance (1), jump in and cross the feet (2). Contract the pelvic floor muscles. Keep knees and feet aligned.	Two beats. Different variations, feet and legpositions.	Rhythm: Jack slow (go low) Jack double tempo Jack syncopated
Jump to wide stance (1), jump in (-and-), jump out (2), jump in (-and-). Or start wide: Jump in (1), out (and), in (2), out (3), hold (4). Position, rhythm, is changed and feet starts/finishes wide.	Two or four beats. A syncopated jumping jack; you jump on and off the beats. Note: In 'Paula Abdul' the torso stays at the same level, only the legs move; out and in.	**Paula Abdul** Jack out; lift/rotate R toe/leg out, lift/rotate L heel in (-and-), jump in (1), jack out; lift/rotate R toe in, lift/rotate L heel/leg out (2), jump in (-and-).
Jump to wide stance (1), stand lift/twist opposite toe and heel out (-and-), back to neutral (2), stand lift/ twist opposite toe and heel out (-and-), to neutral (3), jack in (4). Keep torso level.	Four beats. A syncopated jack with variation. Eight beat variation, e.g.: Jump out (1), hold (2-7) with arm/ torso/leg variation, jump in (8).	Jump out onto heels, toes up, arms up and out (1), rotate legs in/ feet on the floor, cross arms in front (and), rotate legs out, hands on thighs (2), freestyle move (3-6), stand up (7), jumping jack in (8).

JUMP 1

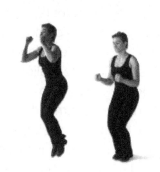

JUMP 2

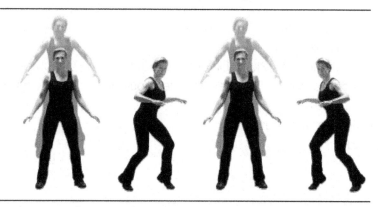

JUMP 3

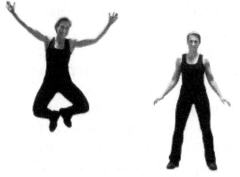

JUMP 4

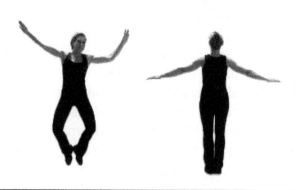

TECHNIQUE	NOTE	VARIATION
Take off from one or both feet, jump, (1) and land on both (2). Feet can land together or apart. Contract the core, stabilize. Neutral step, optimal for transitions.	One or two beats. High and super high impact step. Low and moderate impact; lift up onto your toes. Jumps strengthen the bones, but alternate with low impact steps.	Tempo, Rhythm, Direction ROM (low, high jump) **Jump lift**. Combination of jump and hop with a liftstep. Jump, both feet (1), hop, lift other leg (2); jump curl, skip, knee, kick.
Jump up/down (1), lift the heels/twist both heels right and return (-and-2), jump up/ down (3), lift the heels/ twist both heels left and return (-and-4).	Four beats. Intermediate and advanced level. Keep feet and knees aligned. Jump and twist variation.	Tempo Rhythm Direction Joint movement Amplitude, ROM Arm/upper body movements Style
From wide stance jump up and touch the heels together (1), down, land with feet wide and stand (2). Or repeat. Contract the pelvic muscles during jumps.	Two beats. Advanced level. The leg movement, heels together, requires a certain jump height; take off with power.	Tempo Rhythm Direction Joint movement Amplitude, ROM Arm/upper body movements Style
From wide stance jump up and touch the heels together, at the same time do a ½ turn in the air (1) and land with feet wide (2). Now you are facing the opposite direction.	Two beats. Advanced level. The movement, heels together and a turn, requires a certain jump height; take off with power.	Tempo Rhythm Direction: **Jump turn**, air piruette with a 1/4, 1/2, 1/1, 2/1 turn in the air. Arm/upper body movements Style

DANCE FITNESS STEPS

JOG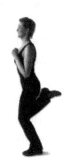

JUMP LUNGE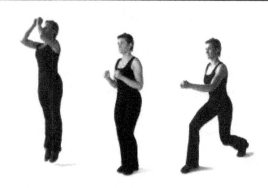

KICK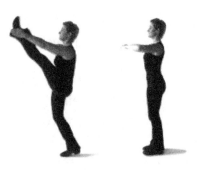

KICK-BALL-CHANGE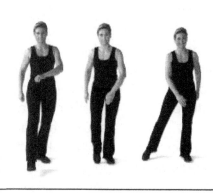

TECHNIQUE	NOTE	VARIATION
Run; take a leap, land on one leg, other leg bends, hamstring curl. Large range of motion, style, heel to buttocks, if desired. Contract the core, stabilize.	One beat. Basic step. High impact. Low impact version is hamstring curl, *not* walk as the joint movement is different. Land toe-ball-heel.	Direction, Travelling Joint movement, ROM Style: **Quebradita step** (ZumbaFitness): Right foot jog in front of left and back. Left foot jog in front of right. Hands in 'the front pockets'; country/cowboy move.
Jump (1) up and land with legs together, jump again and land in lunge position (2). Jump: Take off from all of the foot. Lunge: Land on all of the front foot and on the ball of the back foot.	Two beats. Advanced level. Requires power and practice to stabilize (protect) the knees and feet.	Tempo Rhythm Direction Joint movement Amplitude, ROM Arm/upper body movements Style
Kick with a straight leg (1), lower, bring legs together (2). Or leg behind support leg. Contract the thigh, so the knee is straight throughout the kick. Contract the core, keep the spine neutral.	Two beats. Basic step. **Hitch kick.** Jump up with a bent leg (-and-) and opposite leg kicks, straight leg (1). Land (2). **Scissor kick.** Scissor: Jump and kick (-and-), kick other leg (1). Land (2).	Tempo, Rhythm, Direction, Travelling, Joint movement: **Fan kick (out/in).** Circular kick. Impact, e.g.: **Kick jump**, jump up and kick the leg to the front, side or back.
Kick-support on ball of foot-tap and change (1-and-2): Skip front (1), support on ball of same leg foot (-and-) and tap opposite foot (no weight) to side (2). This changes the lead leg. Repeat/new move.	Two beats. Popular funk, dance and gymnastic step for changing lead leg. Moderate or high impact.	Tempo Direction Travelling Joint movement, plane Amplitude, ROM Arm/upper body movements Style

KNEELIFT

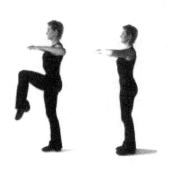 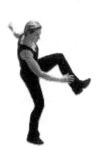

LEAP

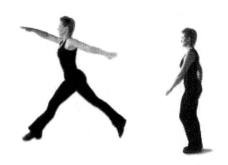

LEG LIFT

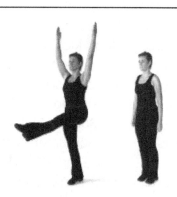

LUNGE (TAP BACK)

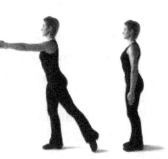

TECHNIQUE	NOTE	VARIATION
Kneelift up (1), legs together (2). *Note: In funk you can contract your abs, 'contraction' in time with the kneelift; stylize.*	Two beats. Base step. Variation, four beats: **Knee cross-over**. Double kneelift, on "2" cross in front, tap. **Knee cross-back.** Double kneelift, on "2" cross behind, tap.	Funky: 1. Walk right 3, pull L knee up, pull R elbow (or both) to the knee and contract "4". 2. Walk right 3, pull L knee up 3 (4-8). Or: Replace middle knee lift with twist "5-and-6".
A running step with a large range of motion: A leap, take off on one foot (1) and land on the other (2).	Two beats. Advanced level. High impact or super high impact step. **Split leap**, sagittal plane. **Frontal split leap** split leap travelling sideways, frontal plane.	Tempo Rhythm Direction Travelling Joint movement Amplitude, ROM Arm/upper body movements Style
Lift the leg approx. 45-90 degrees (1), and lower (2): A low straight leg kick. A full kick ROM is at least shoulder height, in ballet and aer gym approx. 180 degress.	Two beats. Can be a: **Leg Lift Front.** Lift the leg straight in front. **Leg Lift Side.** Lift the leg out (abduction). **Leg Lift Back.** Lift the leg back (10-15 degr.).	Tempo Rhythm Direction Joint movement Amplitude, ROM Arm/upper body movements Impact Style
Extend one leg back, tap (1), return (2). Face forward, diagonal or to the side. Body-weight over working leg. In a side lunge turn the body and legs as one unit; avoid uncontrolled rotation.	Two beats. Base step. Both legs in sagittal plane, no hip rotation. The heel can touch the floor with control, but the bodyweight should stay forward; do not 'fall back'; watch the achilles tendon!	Tempo, Rhythm, Direction Joint: E.g. funky body. Style. Variation: Lunge b (1,2), lunge b (3,4), lunge b/hold foot (5) and twist body back and forth (6,7), legs together (8).

LUNGE

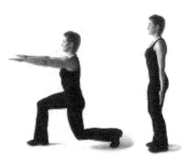

MARCH (WALK)

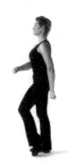

MAMBO (1)

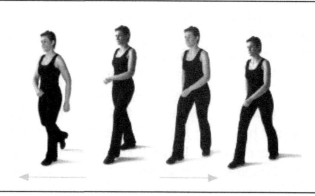

MAMBO (2)

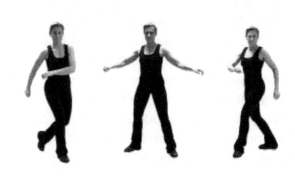

TECHNIQUE	NOTE	VARIATION
A step forward. Both legs bent, back heel is off the floor: Working leg steps forward, moving the center of gravity (1), and steps back, legs together (2).	Two beats. Four beats if using faster music. Contract the thighs, control the movement. Keep knees and feet aligned.	Tempo, Rhythm Direction Joint movement: Front, out, diagonal, back. Amplitude, ROM Upper body movements, e.g. bend torso forward over legs. Style
Number one low impact step (base move). Legs bend, feet move, walk. In fitness: upright torso as in gymnastics. In dance stylize according to music and theme.	One beat. Base step. Numerous variations: Mambo, pivot, step touch, grapevine, V-step, A-step, a.o.	Tempo, Rhythm Direction, Travelling Plane, Joint movement Amplitude Arm/torso movement **Rough neck** (funk): Pull head up and back and release, repeat, during walking. Style
First foot walks forward (1), opposite foot walks in place (2), first foot walks back (3), opposite foot walks in place (4). The body moves with the feet. Walk variation.	Four beats. Popular dance step within many genres, e.g. funk and latin.	Tempo, Rhythm Direction; front, out, back. Arm/upper body moves Impact **Cumbia** (Zumba); mambo double tempo, 1-and-2-and-. Hips out on "1" and "2".
First foot crosses in front (1), second walks on the spot (2), first foot steps out (3), second walks OTS (4). First crosses behind (5), other walks OTS (6), first foot out (7), other OTS (8). Move the body.	Four to sixteen beats. Mambo forward, out or back. Look to the foot. **Multimambo:** Combine front, out, back and front. Style: Drop same side shoulder, when stepping out.	Different tempos: Half (or with double stomp every time), a tempo, or double tempo. Impact Style

DANCE FITNESS STEPS

MAMBO (3)

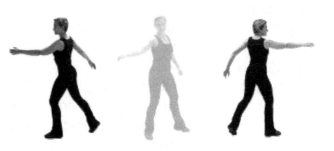

MAMBO (4)

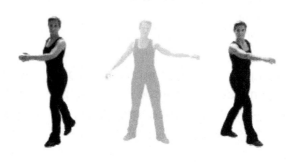

MERENGUE MARCH
(ZumbaFitness©)

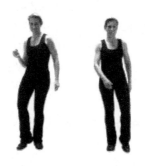

MARCH
BACK AND FORTH

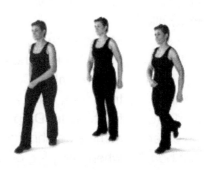

TECHNIQUE	NOTE	VARIATION
1. R Mambo f, chassé (turn ½), mambo L f, chassé (turn ½ to front). 2. R Mambo f, chassé (turn ½), stand, hips RL, chasse turn ½. 3. R Mambo f, chassé (turn ½), pivot ½, walk forward 2.	Eight beats. Mambo with chassé front and back, to front and back wall. Second chassé can be replaced by two walk-steps, to change lead.	In 3. replace the two walk-steps by three quick cross-marches: 4. R Mambo f (1,2), chassé ½ turn to back (3-and-4), pivot ½ (5,6), walk fast and cross feet (7-and-8).
Right foot mambo diagonally in front of left (1,2), chassé right (3-and-4). Left foot mambo in front of right (1,2), chassé back to the left (3-and-4).	Eight beats. Mambo and chassé right and left; in end position add new moves. Variation: Start with chassé and then e.g. mambo behind, R, L.	**Mambo'n'walk** Right foot mambo diagonally in front of left (1,2), chassé right (3-and-4), continue right with four walking steps, while turning, 1/1 or 2/1 turns.
Walk in place. Turn/tip the hip to the support leg side, swing the arms to that side. **Merengue 'pue te mueve'** is two steps right and two steps left with hip and ankle movement.	One beat per step. Walk to latin music with hip, ankle and torso movement; Named Merengue march in Zumba Fitness.	Tempo Direction Travelling Joint movement Amplitude, ROM Arm/upper body movements Impact Style
First foot walks back (1), second foot walks back (2), first foot walks forward (3); or on "1-and-2". Changes lead leg. Walk variation. See Walk variations.	Three beats. When using pop dance music, you need to adjust, e.g. add a hold to fit 4/4.	Tempo Direction Joint movement Amplitude, ROM Arm/upper body movements Impact Style

DANCE FITNESS STEPS

**PADDLE TURN
(TAP TURN)**

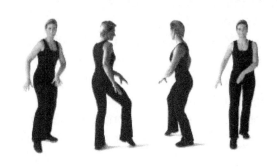

PAS DE BOURRÉ

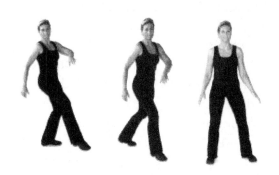

PENDULUM

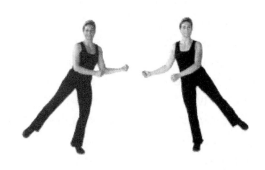

PIROUETTE

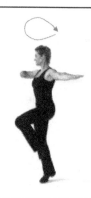

TECHNIQUE	NOTE	VARIATION
Tap/touch one foot on the floor 3-4-8 times, while turning on the supporting leg with the heel lifted. Push or 'paddle' 1/2 or 1/1 turn (4-8 beats).	Four beats. Tap at '12, 9, 6 and 3' o'clock as markers. After the last tap put feet together or continue into a new move.	Tempo Rhythm Direction Joint movement Amplitude, ROM Arm/torso movements Style
Walk/cross first foot behind second foot (1) and second foot walks in place (-and-), first foot return to center (2). Repeat other foot. Walk variation.	Two beats. Three quick steps, behind, in place, out. Ends in demi plié. The torso normally stays centered, as the lead leg 'swings' behind opposite leg.	Tempo Direction Joint movement Amplitude, ROM Arm/torso movements Style
Straight legs swing from side to side as a pendulum. Abduct first leg (1), hop and change leg, abduct second leg (2).	One beat. Two beats; pendulum with both legs. High impact move.	Tempo Rhythm Direction Travelling Joint movement Amplitude, ROM Arm/torso movements Style
A full turn, or more turns, on the ball of one foot. On toes or on the ball of the foot, pivot around the supporting leg. The free leg – and the torso – can be in different positions.	One or two beats. Lift high up onto the ball of the foot. Avoid twisting the knee. Posture, ballet style, should be upright, to make balancing easy.	Tempo Joint movement Amplitude, ROM Arm/torso movements Style: Piruettes with different body positions; modern dance style, more difficult.

DANCE FITNESS STEPS

PIVOT (TURN)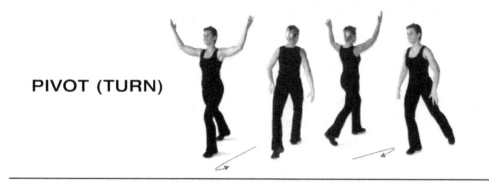

PLIÉ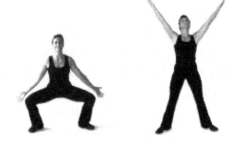

PLIÉ STEP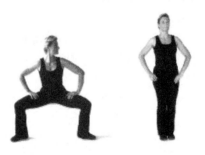

PONY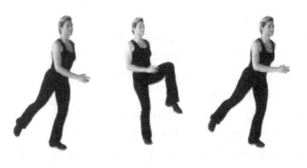

TECHNIQUE	NOTE	VARIATION
A 1/1 turn walk on the spot: First foot walks forward (1), second foot walks in place, turn ½ (2), first foot walks forward (3), second foot walks in place, turn ½ (4).	Four beats. Walk variation. Several variations e.g.: 1. ½ or ¼ turn(s). 2. Pivot without lifting/ moving the second foot: Step forward (1), hold/turn (2), step forward (3), hold/turn (4).	Tempo, Rhythm Direction Joint movement Amplitude Arm and body **Power pivot** 1/1 pivot, end with a jump high in the air. Style
Squat with the feet wide (sumo squat). Bend the legs (1), straighten the legs (2). **Grand plié** is lika a sumo squat with feet wide apart.	Two beats. Contract the pelvic floor muscles. Keep knees and feet aligned. Avoid twisting the knees.	Tempo Rhythm Direction Joint movement Amplitude, ROM Arm/upper body movements Style
Big side step with deep squat, plié (1), feet together (2). You can continue side stepping or step in other directions – or return to the starting position.	Two beats. Contract the pelvic floor muscles. Keep knees and feet aligned. Avoid twisting the knees.	Tempo Rhythm Direction Joint movement Amplitude, ROM Arm/upper body movements Style
Three phases: First leg leaps to the side or forward and lands (1), opposite foot steps in place (2), first leg leaps again (3), either in place or travelling. On the walking step you can lift the knee.	Two beats: Leap and land on "1", change lead on "-and-2". Three beats: With a step on each beat – e.g. with travelling on '1' and '3'. Free leg can perform various movements.	Tempo Direction, Travelling Arm and body Variation: First leg leaps, second extends (1), change legs and do kneelift with the opposite leg (2), leap with first leg again (3).

DANCE FITNESS STEPS

PULL UP

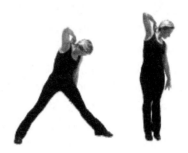

REGGAE
(ZumbaFitness©)

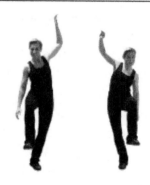

REGGAETON
(ZumbaFitness©)

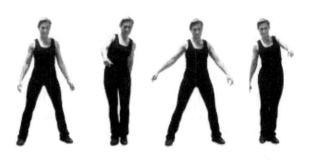

REGGAETON STOMP
(ZumbaFitness©)

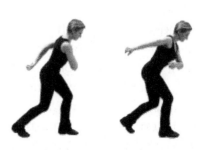

TECHNIQUE	NOTE	VARIATION
Stand. Feet wide. Grab yourself in the neck (collar) (1). 'Pull up' the body; slide the legs in (2).	Two beats. Can be used as an element in a funk or show chroreography.	Tempo Arm/upper body movements Style Can be performed with the arms in other positions.
Stand. Feet shoulder-width apart. Lift R knee/hip, swing/circle left arm back (1,2), lift L knee/hip, swing/circle R arm back (3,4), lift R/L/R knee hold (5-8).	Four or eight beats. Reggae movement.	Tempo Rhythm Direction Amplitude, ROM Arm/upper body movements
Stand. Feet wide. Pull right foot to the left foot and back. Alternate. Rhythm: 1-and, 2-and.	Two beats. A traditional funk step. In ZumbaFitness named Reggaeton.	Tempo Rhythm e.g. and-1, and-2. Direction Arm/upper body movements Style
Stomp forward with the right and left foot alternating, e.g. single, single, double: R, L, R 2. The torso is leaning into the movement and the arms pull to the side, same side as front leg.	Four beats. A lunge type move-ment in which the back leg 'hops' just before changing legs.	Tempo, Rhythm Direction Style **Reggaeton Bounce** Stomp, wide stance, 2 R, 2 L, engage all of the body in the movement.

RELEVÉ

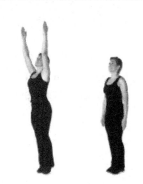

ROCK STEP

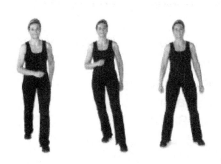

ROCKING HORSE

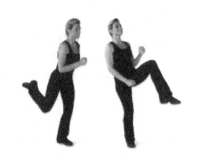

ROGER RABBIT

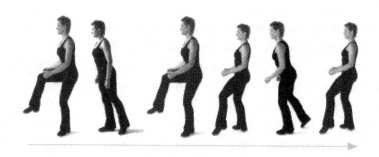

TECHNIQUE	NOTE	VARIATION
A heel raise, up onto the toes (1) and down, lower heels (2).	Two beats. Works well as a moderate impact jump (for beginners). Name is from ballet and modern dance.	Tempo Rhythm Direction Arm/upper body movements Style
First foot step forward, put weight forward (1), step in place with back foot (2), first foot step to the side (3). You can pause in neutral position (4). Repeat opposite. Walk variation.	Three or four beats. Low or moderate impact or high impact.	Tempo Direction Joint movement Amplitude, ROM Arm/upper body movements Impact Style
Feet staggered, in a walk position. First foot steps forward (1), second leg bends, heel to buttocks (2), second foot down (3), first leg makes a kneelift (4).	Four beats. Two beats (gallop): Weight forward on front foot (1), back on back foot (2). Rock back and forth, same foot in front (1,2,1,2,1,2,1,2).	Tempo Rhythm Direction Joint movement Amplitude, ROM Arm/upper body movements Impact Style
First foot steps back, second leg lifts (1), bodyweight rocks forward to front foot (-and-), and back to first foot (2). Second foot steps back (3), etc.	Two beats. Small or large ROM. You can lift the knee or make a small foot movement. During the kneelift, contract the abs; *'contraction'*.	Tempo Direction Travelling Joint movement Amplitude, ROM Arm/upper body movements Style

DANCE FITNESS STEPS

RUNNING MAN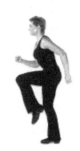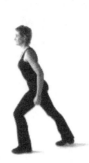

SALSA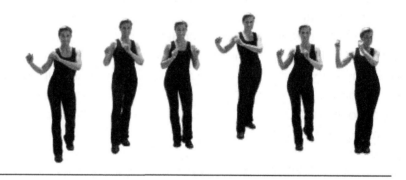

SAMBA (BASIC)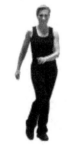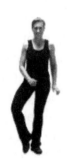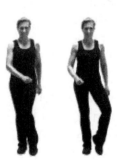

SAMBA LUNGE
(ZumbaFitness©)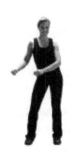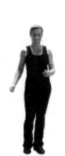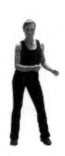

TECHNIQUE	NOTE	VARIATION
Lunge jump with kneelift; rhythm is '1-and- 2-and' or '-and-1- and-2'. Jump; one foot forward, one foot backward (1), lift back knee (-and-). Repeat with opposite leg, ski (2), knee (and).	One and a half beat. After jump: Both feet on the floor or: Weight on front foot, while back foot only touches lightly on the floor. When moving, the foot slides back on the floor in stead of jumping.	Tempo Rhythm Direction Joint movement Amplitude, ROM Arm/upper body movements Impact Style
First foot steps forward and back (1-and-2), second foot back and forward (3-and-4). **Salsa back** Step backward and forward, right and left alternate (1-and-2, 3-and-4)	Four beats. After a sequence with one foot in front; for a balanced fitness workout, perform a sequence with the other foot in front. Body and arms move.	**Cuban salsa** Right mambo out and in (1-and-2), left mambo out (3-and-4). **Salsa travel** Four quick side steps right, 1-and-2-and, four quick side steps left, 3-and-4-and.
Walk in place, rhythm; 1-and, 2-and. Legs rotate in and out. At same time move the hips side to side, small, syncopated movements.	Two beats. Walk with latin style (samba). Requires practice. Walk in place; be on your toes, when the legs 'twist' in and out.	Tempo Rhythm Direction Travelling Arm/upper body movements Style
Take a step out, small side lunge, right, left, and two to the right; R, L, R2. At the same time move the hips side to side.	Four beats. A side lunge in latin style (samba), stylized with torso and hip movement.	Tempo Rhythm Direction Arm/upper body movements Style

SCOOP

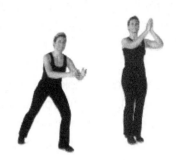

SHIMMY

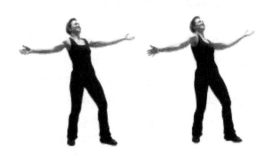

SHUFFLE

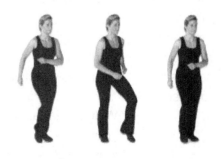

SIDE LUNGE

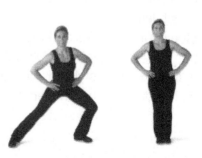

TECHNIQUE	NOTE	VARIATION
As a step touch or step slide with a jump: Step (1), jump/feet together (2).	Two beats. Step touch in moderate or high impact	Tempo Rhythm Direction Travelling Joint movement Amplitude, ROM Arm/upper body movements Style
Stand. Feet wide. Shake the shoulders back and forth, fast tempo.	One or more beats. Learn by practicing a tempo to music, then double tempo, then faster.	Tempo Rhythm Style Add torso movement, e.g. by leaning backward and forward.
Low impact jog in double tempo with travelling, 1-and, 2-and, 3-and, 4-and. Same leg starts every time.	Four beats. Travelling, short or longer distances.	Tempo Rhythm Direction Travelling Joint movement Amplitude, ROM Arm/upper body movements Style
Large lunge to side. First leg steps out, land with bent knee (1), other leg is straight and relaxed. Weight is on the lunging leg. Push off and return, legs together (2). Or stay and add a new move.	Two beats. Watch the knees. **Stationary sidelunge** Feet super wide, shift weight; side to side. **Stationary lunge 1/1/2** R/L/R (hold), torso/arm move on '3-and-4'.	1. Sidelunge R, L, R2. Press arms opposite. 2. Sidelunge O/I 3 (1-6), jump center 2 (turn 1/1) (7,8). 3. Sidelunge O/I 3, on middle lunge turn body 1/4 or ½ and turn back, return.

DANCE FITNESS STEPS

SKATE

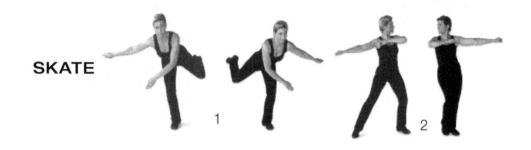

1   2

SKIING (SCISSORS)

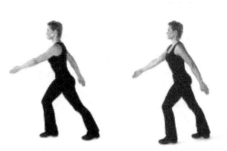

SKI JUMP (SIDE JUMP)

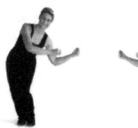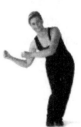

SKIP

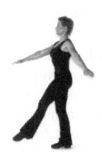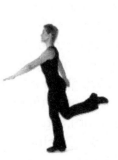

TECHNIQUE	NOTE	VARIATION
1: Step hamstring curl (1, 2), leaning forward and swing the arms from side to side as a skater. 2: Step touch with 'attitude': Face in the step direction and swing arms opposite.	Two beats. Low impact step. Intermediate level: A forward lean requires core control; stabilize to protect the back. Limit the number of repetitions.	Tempo, Rhythm Direction, Travelling Variation: 1. Double tempo skate. 2. Wide stance, pull one foot to the other and back (-and-1) and repeat with the opposite foot (-and-2).
Jump, land with feet staggered; one foot in front, one foot back (1), jump and change legs, so opposite leg now is in front (2). Alternate.	One or two beats. A single 'skiing' jump can be used as a transition; land with staggered feet. From here e.g. turn ¼ and continue into jumping jack 'in'.	Tempo Rhythm Direction Style Variation: Between each jump, jump into legs together position, before jumping and changing legs.
Jump, legs together, from side to side. Jump right (1), jump left (2). You can perform an extra jump ('pause'); jump right (1), jump in place (2), jump left (3), jump in place (4).	One beat. Two beats to return. Intermediate to advanced level. Contract the core, pelvic floor muscles and leg muscles well. Land with soft knees. High impact move.	Tempo Direction Joint movement Amplitude, ROM Arm/upper body movements Style
Low kick from bent to straight knee. High impact: Hop, bend the leg (prepare) (1), and skip (2). Low impact: Skip (1) and legs together (2). Contract the quads to control the movement.	Two beats. Basic step. Funky variation: **Wiping off shoes** Curl leg back, kick forward and slide the shoe across the floor as to wipe off dirt. Variation: Perform the wipe the opposite way.	Tempo, Rhythm Direction, Travelling **Combat kick** Front kick, Side kick and Back kick **Andale step** (Zumba) First leg kneelift (1,2), other leg swing/kick behind (3,4).

DANCE FITNESS STEPS

SLIDE (STEP)

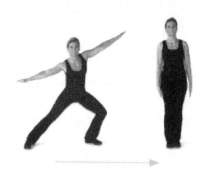

SQUAT

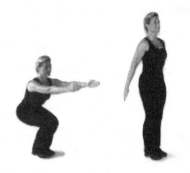

STEP CURL

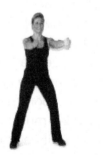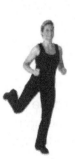

STEP OUT JACK

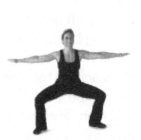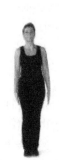

TECHNIQUE	NOTE	VARIATION
Gliding or sliding. A long, dragging step touch: First foot takes a large side step (1), the other foot slides to it, legs together (2). Often in half or slow tempo for longer and 'softer' steps.	Two beats. Watch the knees during wide side and slide steps. Perform with control.	Tempo, Rhythm 1. Slide to side (1,2), stand, torso movements (3-and-4-and-). 2. Slide to side (1,2), stand and twist (3-and-4). 3. Slide to the side (1,2), feet together, move the hips (3-4).
Legs together, hip- or shoulder-width apart or wide. Bend the legs, go down (1). Extend the legs, return up (2).	Two beats. Neutral step, nice for transitions. Add style. Limit the number of squats in a series, max. 1-4, to keep the dance style. Avoid endurance work.	Tempo, Rhythm Direction Joint movement, ROM Arm/upper body movements Style: Squats are made funky by using the torso and the feet.
First leg step to the side (1), second leg hamstring curl, heel to buttocks (2). The curl is on "2", different from leg curl (on "1"). Step touch variation.	Two beats. Can be stylized in numerous ways; hand to foot, upper body movements, half tempo lifts or holds or piruette on the lift.	Tempo Rhythm Direction, Travelling Joint movement Amplitude, ROM Arm/upper body movements Impact Style
A low impact jumping jack. From feet together position, step out into wide squat (1), both legs bent (as opposed to sidelunge). Step back in, legs together (2).	Two beats. Contract the pelvic floor muscles. Watch the knee during lateral movements. Also called **half jack** or **squat side**.	Tempo Rhythm Direction Joint movement Amplitude, ROM Arm/upper body movements Style

STEP TOUCH (1)

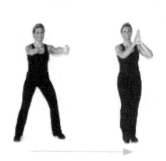

STEP TOUCH (2)

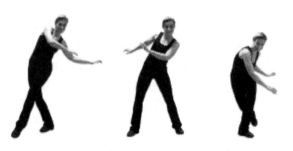

STEP TOUCH (3)

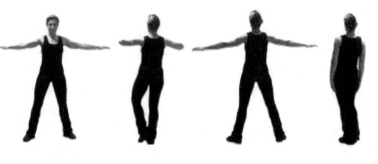

STEP TOUCH (4)

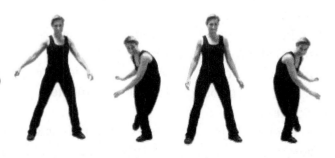

TECHNIQUE	NOTE	VARIATION
First leg steps to the side (1), second foot closes, taps lightly (2). Walk variation. You can also side step and step together; a walk two. And continue in the same direction in stead of going back.	Two beats. **Double step touch** Even if it is called so and is built from step touch, it is a combo of walking three steps to the side and a single touch, tap.	Tempo, Rhythm Direction, Travelling Plane (fx front/back) Arms and body Style, e.g.: **Cumbia candle** (Zumba) Double step touch, R and L, one hand lifted as holding a candle.
First leg steps to the side (1), second foot taps in front or behind (2). The body leans into the movement. **Step touch stomp** For every step, do a double stomp: Step R (1-and), together (2-and).	Two beats. An easy funk step. Contract the muscles of the supporting leg well to stabilize and protect the knee. Don't stomp too hard.	Tempo, Rhythm Direction, Travelling Arms and upper body Style, e.g. accentuated downward-movement; step out and 'fall down', go up again. Repeat.
Step touch with half turn (2 x ½ turn): Step touch R, turn ½ (1,2), step touch L (3,4). Step touch R, turn ½ (5,6), step touch L (7,8).	Eight beats. Can also be done as a 'corner'; Step touch R/L (1-4), turn 1/4 and step touch R/L (5-8), turn 1/4 back. Can be performen in a U-pattern turning first right, then left (2 x 8).	Tempo Direction Travelling Arm/upper body movements Style
Step touch combo: Step touch R (1), L tap behind (2), step touch L (3), R tap behind (4), step wide, stand (5), jump and land with R crossed in front of L, slowly turn 1/1 (7,8).	Eight beats. Variations: Tap front or behind. Step touch combos with turns. You can change tempo, direction, travelling and torso movements.	Step touch R (1), L tap behind (2), step touch L (3), R tap behind (4), step touch R (5), L tap behind (6), step touch L (7), R tap behind and turn ½ or 1/1 (8),

DANCE FITNESS STEPS

STEP TOUCH POWER

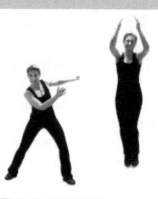

STOMP

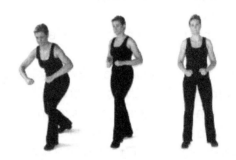

STROLL

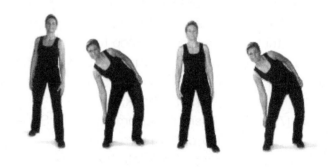

SWANK

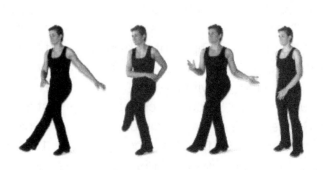

TECHNIQUE	NOTE	VARIATION
Step touch in high impact: **Step jump** First foot step to the side (1), jump on both feet and close legs (2).	Two beats. Arm/torso movements styled to match the music. E.g. large arm circles with both arms or alternate.	Tempo Rhythm Direction Travelling Joint movement Amplitude, ROM Arm/upper body movements Style
Push your foot into the floor. E.g.: Step forward and push the foot into the floor (1), walk in place with second foot (2), step back with first foot (3), etc. Walk variation.	One, two or three beats. Often a series of eight beats; stomp with right and left foot, different rhythms. Stomp with just one foot for a number of repetitions.	Tempo Rhythm Direction Travelling Joint movement Amplitude, ROM Arm/upper body movements Style
Walk forward 4, legs wide and bent (1-4). Torso, shoulder and arm lean into the movement. Accent on beat '2' and '4', go deeper. Walk back in the same way (5-8). Walk variation.	Four beats. Eight beats forward and back. After a 'set', repeat with the other leg. Low impact step. The style is funky.	Tempo Direction Travelling Joint movement Amplitude, ROM Arm/upper body movements
First leg skips forward twice. After the first skip (1), bend the knee, lower leg in front of opposite leg (-and-), skip forward again (2). Legs together (3,4) or another move.	Four beats. Double skip. Leg skips twice (1,2), legs together, hold (3,4). Several styles, a.o. funk and latin.	Tempo Direction Joint movement Amplitude, ROM Arm/upper body movements Style: Stylize to the music, with or without jumping.

STAND (1)
and …

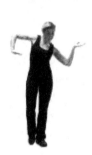

STAND (2)
and …

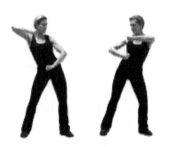

STAND (3)
and …

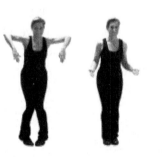 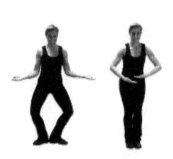

STAND (4)
and …

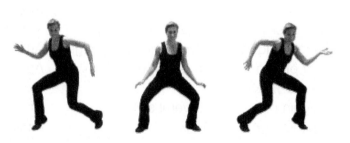

TECHNIQUE	NOTE	VARIATION
Standing on the spot. Perform arm, torso and leg variations without travelling (moving). *Note: If the goal is a cardio workout: Avoid standing too long in one place, normally max. eight beats.*	One or more beats. Variation: Bodycircles, waves, shoulder rolls, up/down, front/back. **Bodywave.** Go up and down and up: Lift heels, lower heels, bend knees, continue wave up, joint by joint.	**Pop** Sharp movements with 'contraction', as a robot; breakdance. **Snake (worm)** Isolated body ripples, isolations. Standing or while travelling.
Standing on the spot. Upper body move to the side without moving the legs, 'waist press'. *Note: If the goal is a cardio workout: Avoid standing too long in one place, normally max. eight beats.*	One or more beats. **Robocop** Feet wide. Upper body, shoulders level, move right and left, 1/1/2. Pull the elbow to the side, as if you pull a rope.	**Bodyroll side.** Step out, lean body and head into movement; *as if entering through a small window sideways,* then turn body ¼, pull in shoulders and turn ¼ back, move body sideways in and up.
Stand, rotate feet out and in. You can travel or turn to the side. 1. Rotate the legs (heels) out/in, pull the elbows up/down at the same time. 2. Rotate legs (toes) out/in, forearms out/in.	One or more beats. Feet can point 1) in same direction 2) towards each other 3) away from each other At the same time or alternatingly. Travelling.	**Bodyroll** (quebradita, Zumba). Circle FUBD: Stand. Feet staggered front/back. Lean all of the body forward, stick the chest out (1), lean back, hips forward (-and-), bend the legs, weight on back leg (2).
Stand. Lift/rotate right left out and lift/rotate left leg in (1), return to centre, lower heels (-and-), lift/rotate right leg in and lift/rotate left leg in (2), return to centre (-and-).	One or more beats. Turn legs, hip rotation and lift up onto either 1) the balls of the feet, 2) the heels or 3) heel and ball of the foot.	Stand. Lift/rotate R leg out, lift toes, lift/rotate L leg in, lift heel (1), return to centre, lower feet (-and-), lift/rotate R leg in, lift heel, lift/ rotate L leg out, lift toes, (2), return to center (-and-).

TAP (1)

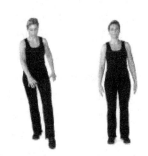

TAP (2) and ...

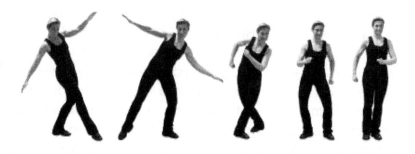

TAP (3) and ...

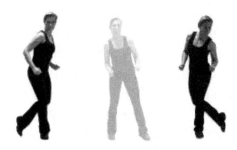

TAP (4) and ...

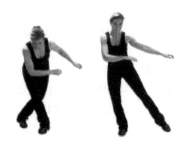

TECHNIQUE	NOTE	VARIATION
Toe tap or heel dig front, back or out (1), feet (close) together (2). Instead of closing the feet lift the knee. **Cross front**. Tap in front of the other foot. **Cross back**. Tap behind the other foot.	Two beats. One beat if double tempo jump tap: Toe tap (1), jump, change foot (2). Tap is a non-weight-bearing step. Cross front or back is best with feet wide.	**Tobago** (Zumba): Tap R toe out (1), tap R heel forward (2), jump change. Tap L toe out (3), tap L heel forward (4), jump change. Arm/torso movement Style
Tap R foot in front of L (1), tap R foot out to the side (2), R foot walk/step behind L (3), walk two in place, double tempo (-og-4): **Tap and cross back.** Repeat with the other foot.	Two beats. One beat if double tempo jump tap: Toe tap (1), jump, change foot (2).	Tempo, Rhythm Direction, Travelling Style: Tap forward, hips forward, lean torso back, arms over the head (1), legs together, arms down and back (2).
Tap R behind L (1), out and hold (2), tap L behind R (3), out and hold (4), tap R behind L (5), walk three and turn 1/1 backwards to the right (6,7,8). Repeat left. **Tap and turn.**	Two beats. One beat if double tempo jump tap: Toe tap (1), jump, change foot (2).	Tempo Rhythm Direction Joint movement Amplitude Arm/torso movement Style
1. Walk R F, tap L out, walk L F, tap R out, etc. 2. Walk three forward, cross the feet, R/L/R, tap L out "4", walk three forward cross the feet, L/R/L, tap R foot out "8". **Walk and tap.**	Two or more beats. Combination of walk and tap; walk or walk crossing the feet and tap out (side touch).	Tempo Rhythm Direction Travelling Joint movement Amplitude Arm/torso movement Style

TOE TOUCH

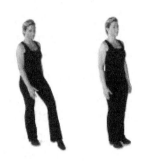

**TOUCH OUT
(SIDE TOUCH)**

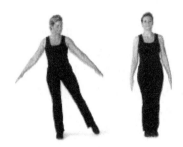

TRIPLET

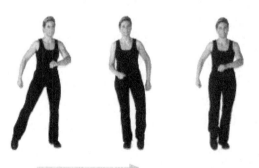

TRIPPLE STEP

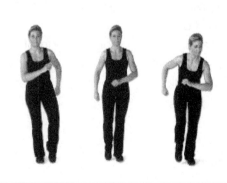

TECHNIQUE	NOTE	VARIATION
Tap toes (ball of foot) (1), feet together (2). Variation: Tap alternatingly or tap twice with right and left followed by a pause of two. Or tap three, feet together (4) and repeat.	Two beats. **Toe Touch Front** (Push Touch Front). Tap toes in front of other leg. **Toe Touch Back** (or Push Touch Back). Tap toes back/behind. **Toe Touch Side** (as Touch Out), to the side.	Tempo Direction Joing movement Amplitude Arm/torso movement Style
Keep the body weight centered, while the foot taps to the side (1) and back to center position (2). Repeat or repeat with the other leg.	Two beats. Do combinations, e.g. tap front (1), out (2), back (3), together (4), with torso movement. Repeat with the other leg.	Tempo, Rhythm Direction, Travelling Arm/torso movement **Touch out three** R out (1), in (-and-), L out (2), in (-and-), R out (3), lift R knee fast (-and-), R foot down (4). Repeat other foot.
Three-part step on '1-and-2'. Accent on "1", "and" or "2". E.g. as a step touch, the rhythm '1-and-2'. One foot out (1), other foot closes (-and-), weight on first foot (2).	Two beats. Walk variation. Can be a low impact step or a bouncy moderate impact step or high impact with hops.	Tempo Rhythm Direction, Travelling Joint movement Amplitude Arm/torso movement Impact Style
Three-part march or jog on '1-and 2'. Accent on "2". You can lift the knee on "2". Rhythm: A tempo, a tempo, hold/stick. Walk variation.	Two beats. Can be performed with a longer hold, so move lasts four beats. Stylize with more or less upper body movement.	Tempo Rhythm Direction, Travelling Joint movement Amplitude Arm/torso movement Impact Style

TUCK JUMP

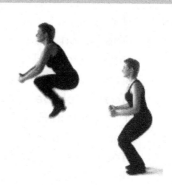

TWIST

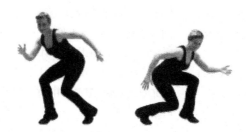

TWIST JUMP

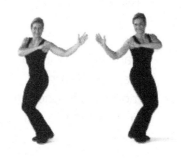

V-STEP

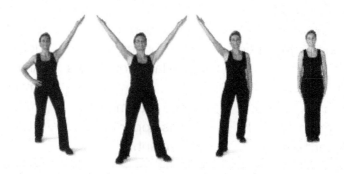

TECHNIQUE	NOTE	VARIATION
Jump high. Pull the knees towards your chest, thighs above horizontal (1). Land with the feet together (2). Variation: Land with the feet apart.	Two beats. For intermediate to advanced exercisers. High or super high impact move. Contract the core. Controlled landing.	Tempo, Rhythm Direction Joint movement Amplitude Arm/torso movement **Frog jump** Same type of jump, but lower and with the legs apart.
Twist, turn from side to side. Legs together or apart. Variation: Twist and kneelift, e.g. twist R/L/R, kneelift L, twist L/R/L, kneelift R.	One or two beats. Low impact. Lift the heels, when twisting and twist on the balls of the feet. Contract the thigh muscles to stabilize the knees. And/or keep legs together.	Tempo, Rhythm Direction, Travelling Plane/level (low, high), e.g. twist down, up. Arm/torso movement Style
Twist jump, turn from side to side. Legs together or apart. A neutral step with the legs close together and body weight distributed evenly across the feet.	One or two beats. High impact. Knees and feet aligned; contract the thigh muscles to stabilize the knees. Press inner thighs together during twists for increased stability.	Tempo, Rhythm Direction, Travelling Plane/level (low, high), e.g. twist down, up. ROM 45-180 degr. Arm/upper body movements Style
Legs steps out in a V: First foot forward and out (1), second fod forward and out (2) (legs wide), first foot steps back and in, second foot back and in (4), feet together. A walk variation.	Four beats. Two if double tempo. Variation: Reverse V (also called A-step): Step back out, out, step forward, in, in, feet together or lift step to change lead.	Tempo Rhythm Direction Joint movement Amplitude Arm/torso movement Impact Style

DANCE FITNESS STEPS

WALK (MARCH) 1
and ...

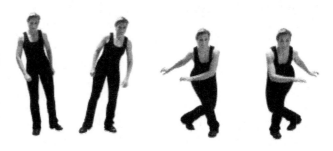

WALK (MARCH) 2
and ...

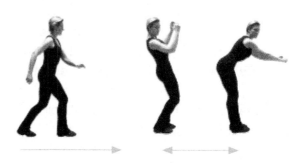

WALK (MARCH) 3
and ...

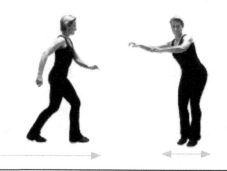

WALK (MARCH) 4
and ...

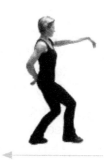

TECHNIQUE	NOTE	VARIATION
1a. Walk in place (funky) 3, tap/kick leg out. 1b. Walk sideways 3, kick leg to the side. 1c. Syncopated walk (1-and-2) and kick leg out twice (3,4).	Four beats. Walk and lift combos: walk (1), kick – or tap – other leg front, out or back (2), walk 2 (3, 4).	Tempo, Rhythm, Direction, Travel Joint movement, e.g.: Bent legs or on toes. **Cross walk**: Walk and cross in front, on the spot or travelling. Arm/upper body moves, Style
2a. Walk right 1,2, jump 2 (3,4) right. Or: Walk 3, jump 1. Walk 4, jump 4. 2b. Walk right 1,2, jump forward and back (3-and-4). Repeat left. 2c. Walk right 1,2, jump forward 3 (3-and-4).	Four beats. Walk combination; walk is combined with jumps or slides. For four or more beats.	Tempo, Rhythm Direction, Travelling Joint movement Amplitude Arm/upper body movements Impact Style
3a. Walk right 3, twist (-and-4). 3b. Walk right 3, stand, rotate left leg out, point left arm out, circle right arm over the head "4". 3c. Walk right 3, stand, cross your arms and circle the arms "4".	Four beats. Walk combinations; walk is combined with a stationary movement, e.g. standing or twisting on the spot.	Walk right 3, stand and lift L hip/heel and put R arm forward, lift R hip/heel and put L arm forward, lift L hip/heel and put R arm forward.
Walk backwards three to the right (1-3), turn ½ on "4". Repeat to return. Add upper body movements, e.g. one arm, straight or bent, in front of the torso.	Four beats. Walk variation with upper body moves and travelling.	Tempo, Rhythm Travelling, Style Joint movement, e.g.: Walk like an **Egyptian** Walk with bent legs, the head moves back and forth. Arms make egyptian movements.

DANCE FITNESS STEPS

WALK, 'STAGGER'

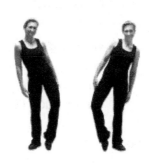

WALK, 'STUMBLE'

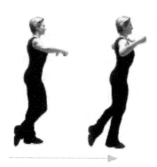

WALK, 'SLOW MOTION'

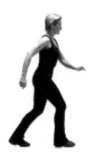

WALK, 'SHAKE IT OUT'

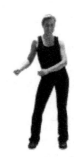

TECHNIQUE	NOTE	VARIATION
Walk in place, 'sway': Turn the legs out, hip external rotation, walk with right and left foot alternating; 'Fall' out on the entire foot and straight leg, relax, bend, opposite leg and touch toes to floor.	One beat. Two beats, when left and right leg walks. Low impact step. Body sways or rocks from side to side.	Tempo Rhythm Direction Travelling Amplitude Arm/upper body movements Style
Walk forward, e.g. 4 or 8 steps. For every step 'fall' forward with body, so back foot 'stumbles' on the floor; top of the foot touches the floor. Shoulders and arms can circle forward.	One beat. Two beats, when left and right leg walks. Low impact step. Avoid load (body-weight) on the 'stumbling' ankle.	Tempo Rhythm Direction Arm/torso movements Style
Walk in place or travelling in different different directions. Move all of the body slowly; slow motion movement.	Four or more beats. Low impact. Stylize with arm and torso movements. Super slow motion; tai chi style moves.	Tempo Direction Travelling Joint movement Amplitude Arm/torso movements Style
Walk in place or travelling in different different directions. Shake the head, arms, hands, hips, legs and feet.	One or two beats. Walking with 'shaking' movements is an easy way for beginners to get into 'freestyle'. To 'shake it out' feels nice for new as well as advanced dancers.	Tempo Rhythm Direction Travelling Joint movement Amplitude Arm/torso movements Style

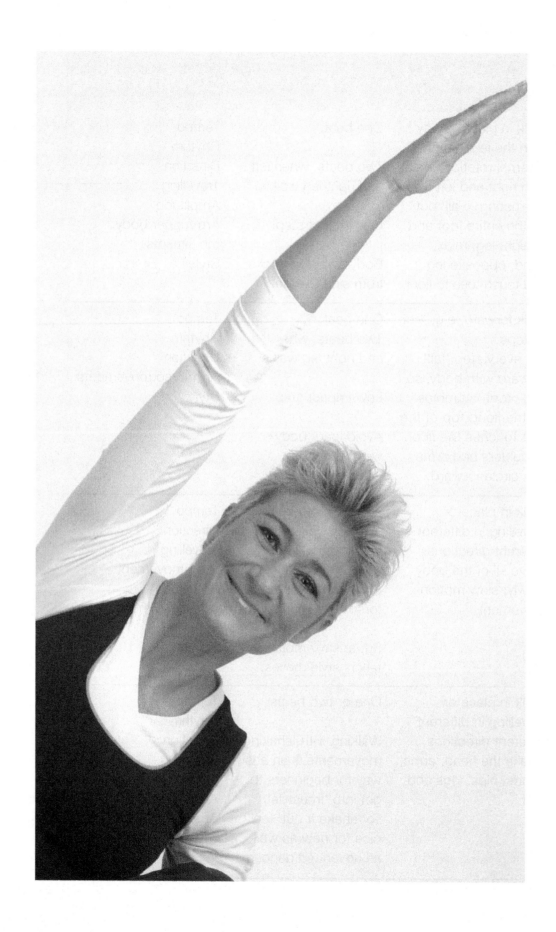

Appendix | **Upper body moves**

The next two pages show all the fundamental upper body movements.
The table covers the main exercises for most major muscle groups.

These movements can be used as shown for easy, basic upper body work. However, they are also included in order to inspire instructors to develop their own unique upper body exercises.

The movements can be styled in numerous ways, using one or both arms and with the torso in different positions. You can create new moves to different music genres.

Most of the moves or exercises are depicted as bilateral moves, moves with both arms working at the same time and in symmetry, which is easier for beginners.
Most moves can also be performed as unilateral moves; with one arm only, which is also easy for beginners. Or in combinations or mixed asymmetric movements for experienced exercisers.

Note: The table uses general names from dance and fitness.
They can be replaced or complemented by images such as 'embrace', 'whip' 'shake', 'wave etc.

DANCE FITNESS UPPER MODY MOVES

Head/neck	Turn, right, left Half circle, right, left	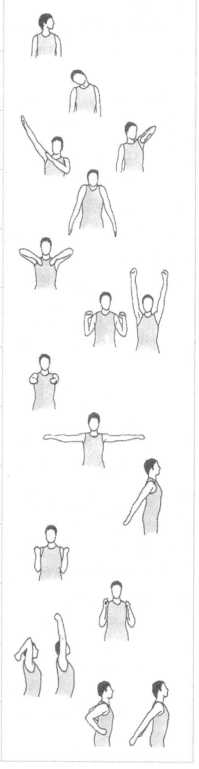
Neck	Sidebend, right, left Bend, extend	
Shoulder circles	Half, full circle, swing Rotation in/out (low/high) with straight/bent arms	
Shoulder raises (shrugs)	Shrug the shoulder(s); lift and lower the shoulders	
Upright row	Lift elbows above horizontal. Hands follow, stop under the chin.	
Shoulder press	Press the arms up to vertical position and lower. Variation: Rotation.	
Front raise	Lift the arms forward to horizontal. Variation: High front raise to vertical.	
Side (lateral) raise	Lift arms out to the side, to horizontal. Add: Turn palms up and continue upwards.	
Extension (pullback)	Lift arms straight back. Straight or bent arms.	
Biceps curl	Bend the arms (elbows). Variation: Different planes, e.g. externally rotated.	
Hammer curl	Bend the arms. Palms face each other, thumbs up.	
Triceps extension	Extend (and bend) elbows. Arms in vertical position.	
Triceps press	Extend (and bend) elbows. Arms up, out or back.	

DANCE FITNESS UPPER BODY MOVES

Torso movements	Bend, extend, sidebend right, left, rotate right, left	
Fly	Adduct the arms in front of the body. Arms bent or straight, different angles.	
Chest cross (cross)	Cross the arms in front of the body. Arms bent or straight, different angles.	
Press (chest press)	Push the arms forward in front of body, horizontal plane (and pull back).	
Push (jab/punch)	Punch forward. Punch up, straight forward or down.	
Swing (hook/uppercut)	Swing in front of body. Hook: Towards temple. Uppercut: Towards jaw.	
Lat pull (pulldown)	Pull the arms down or back from above or front of the body.	
Row (rowing)	Pull the arms back. Elbows out (rhomboid) or straight back (latissimus).	
Speedball	Roll the forearms around each other. Slow, a tempo, fast or super fast.	
Hand movements	Wrists neutral or bent. Fingers together or apart, straight or bent. Clap and snap.	

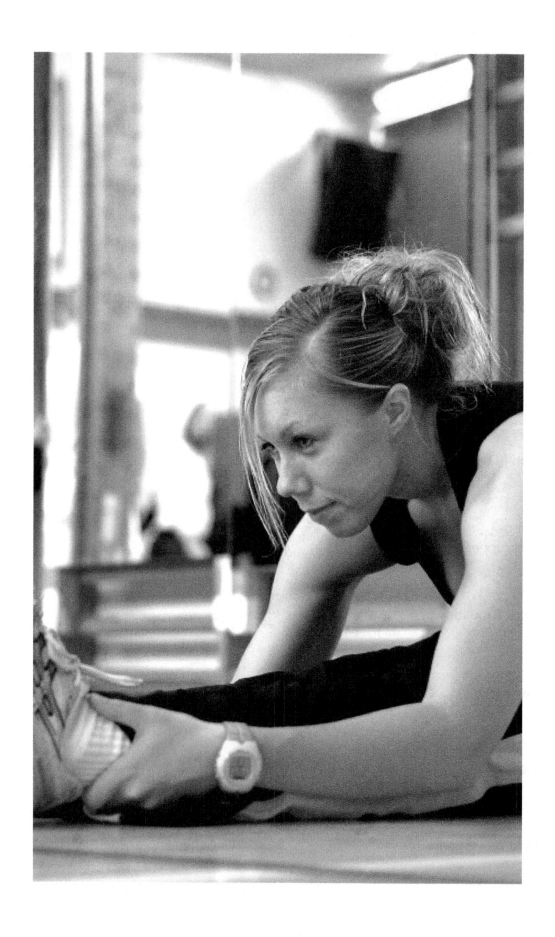

Appendix | **Dance stretches**

The next three pages has an overview of dance and dance fitness stretches.

The first guide covers stretches for beginners: Easy traditional fitness stretches for the major muscles.
These stretches can be performed by almost all exercisers and are for all-round flexibility.

The next two guides are for intermediate and advanced level dancers. Some of these stretches requires a certain degree of initial flexibility.

Note: Dance fitness does not require, that you are flexible. Actually too much mobility can result in too little stability.
However, for some dances and shows you need to be quite flexible.

The stretches are in the order of hip and leg stretches first; if you only have limited time for stretching, prioritize calves, hamstrings and hip flexors, as these muscles are tight in many people.

Note: Exercisers differ in flexibility, so each stretch should be adapted to suit individual needs.

A certain mobility of the spine is important: You should include flexion, extension, lateral flexion and rotation in warm-ups and cooldowns.

Hold cooldown stretches for 20-60 seconds for general flexibility.
For extra flexibility, e.g. for splits, warm-up and hold the stretches for up to 2-5 minutes.

Dance fitness stretches, beginners

Shins (ankle mobility, uphold stability)	Standing. Legs parallel, hip-width apart and staggered. Top of the back foot on the floor. Gently stretch across the ankle.	
Calves	Standing. Legs parallel, hip-width apart and staggered, large step. Back heel on the floor. Back leg knee straight, then bent.	
Calves **Hip flexor**	Standing. Legs parallel, hip-width apart and staggered, slightly bent. Calf stretch: Keep back heel down. Hip flexor stretch: Move back leg further back. Contract abs and buttocks.	
Hamstrings	Standing. Legs parallel, hip-width apart and staggered. Weight on back foot. Neutral spine. Arms support on back leg. Front leg knee straight. Buttocks back. (Dorsi)flex the foot to stretch the calf.	
Adductors	Standing. Legs wide and externally rotated; knees and toes out; aligned. Bend legs. Arms on the inside of thighs, push lightly outward.	
Abductors	Standing with legs close. One leg behind the other. Push the hips out to the side of the back leg. Lean the torso opposite.	
Quads (thighs) **Hip flexor**	Standing. Legs close, no hip-rotation. Bend one leg, grab ankle with one or both hands. Hip forward, knee behind support leg. Contract abs and buttocks.	
Buttocks	Sitting (or standing). One leg crossed over the other. Pull the top leg towards the body until you feel a stretch in the deep buttock muscles (piriformis). Bottom leg bent or straight.	

Table: Dance fitness stretches for beginners.

Dance fitness stretches, beginners

Lower back (spinal mobility, uphold stability)	On all fours. Light support on the hands, arms straight. Bend; hunch the back. Tuck the pelvis under, pull the tailbone down. *Do not overdo back stretching as stability is of primary importance.*	
Upper back	Kneeling. Upper body forward. Arms forward, palms on the floor. Push the hands down and pull the body away from hands. Move one arm across the other, lean slightly in to the shoulder of top arm.	
Upper back	Kneeling. Hands together. Arms forward in front of the body in horizontal plane. Pull the arms forward and abduct the shoulder blades for a back side stretch.	
Abdominals	Prone. Support on the forearms. (If you are very flexible, support on your hands with arms straight, hands below shoulders). Push forearms down and try to move torso forward, stretch the abs.	
Chest, shoulder and arm, front	Kneeling. Upper body leans forward. Arms to the side, palms to the floor. Bend one arm and turn the torso towards it. The other forearm remains on the floor, push shoulder gently down; stretch.	
Shoulder, middle part	Kneeling. Move the arm to be stretched behind the body. Opposite hand pulls gently at the forearm. Sidebend head (neck) to the side of the pulling arm.	
Arm, back (triceps)	Kneeling. Hold one arm (to be stretched) vertical, bend the elbow and move hand towards shoulder blade. The other hand pushes gently on the elbow to increase the stretch.	
Forearms	On all fours. Palms on the floor, turn the fingers towards the legs. Keep the weight on the legs, do not over-load (bodyweight) the arms and hands. Gentle forearm stretch.	

Table: Dance fitness stretches for beginners.

Dance fitness stretches, intermediate

Ankles and feet	Standing. Lift the heel of the working leg, light support on toes. Make circles with the working leg, circle both ways.	
Calves	Standing. Feet hip-width apart. Heels and hands on the floor. Body in yoga 'dog position'. Bend one leg and stretch opposite leg calf muscles.	
Hamstrings Hip flexors	Kneeling. Kneel down, one foot forward, one back. Slide front leg forward and slide into sagittal split position.	
Adductors	Prone in frog position. Bent legs turned out. Lower legs, inner thighs on floor. Watch the knees.	
Quads (thighs)	Kneeling. One foot forward, knee above foot. Other leg bent, support on thigh (above knee), grab ankle, bend the knee.	
Buttocks (glutes)	Sitting. Drop left bent leg to the side. Right leg bent, foot in front of left lower leg. Lean forward, head to left knee.	
Abs (torso)	Kneeling. Bend backwards as in a bridge. Hands grab hold of the ankles for support.	
Upper back Shoulders	Kneeling (or standing). Lean forward. Support the arms on the floor or a wall; move the torso down to stretch.	
Shoulder Neck	Both arms behind the torso. One hand holds opposite elbow and pulls at that arm. Head turns away and looks down.	
Chest	Standing. In doorway. Both arms to the side and lean gently forward. Or hand on wall or bar. Press gently to stretch.	
Shoulder, arm	Sitting. Palms on the floor behind the body. Slide away from hands; increase distance between hands and buttocks.	
Arm, back	One arm vertical, bend the arm behind the body. Bend opposite arm behind. Let fingers grab each other. Pull gently.	

Table: Dance fitness stretches, intermediate level. Including selected exercises/drawings adapted/redrawn from 'Sports Stretches' by Alter published by Human Kinetics.

Dance fitness stretches, advanced

Ankles and feet	Standing. Lift the heel of the working leg, light support on toes. Make circles with the working leg, circle both ways.	
Calves	Standing, 5. position. Legs out. Feet in front/behind each other, heels by toes. Stand with straight legs and bent legs.	
Hamstrings Hip flexors	Sitting; sagittal split. Both legs straight. One forward, one back, no hip rotation. Watch the knees. Hands can support.	
Adductors	Sitting; frontal split, legs to the side. 180 degr. split. Upper body (abs) on the floor; 'pancake'. Watch the knees.	
Quads (thighs)	Sitting; sagittal split. Bend back leg, lower leg vertical. Bend backward and grab the ankle with the hands.	
Buttocks (glutes)	Standing. Lift, bend, externally rotate one leg and put it on a bar or table. Lean forward to increase the stretch.	
Abs (torso)	Bridge position. Feet on the floor, together or apart. Hands on the floor, fingers point to feet.	
Upper back Shoulders	Standing. Upper body leans forward. Rest the hands on a wall or a bar; move the torso further down to stretch.	
Shoulder Neck	Supine, yoga 'plough' position. Support on the shoulders, not the neck. Bend the legs, drop lower legs to the floor.	
Chest	Standing. In doorway. Both arms to the side and lean gently forward. Or hands on wall or bar. Press gently to stretch.	
Shoulder, arm	Standing. Bend the arms and put the palms together behind the body.	
Arm, back	One arm vertical, bend the arm behind the body. Bend opposite arm behind. Let fingers grab each other. Pull gently.	

Table: Dance fitness stretches, advanced level. Including selected exercises/drawings adapted/redrawn from 'Sports Stretches' by Alter published by Human Kinetics.

Appendix | **Dance notation**

On the next page there is an example of verse-chorus choreography notes; the beats of the music and structure.

Artist, title, duration and tempo, beats per minute, BPM, are listed.

The beats are grouped in 'eight-counts' and 'blocks' to show the music, song, structure.

On the basis of the music analysis the base choreography is made.

During the first listenings, the basic moves, steps, are tested to find the ones best suited.

The base moves are noted (for later, more choreography work).

Note: It is not necessary to write '4 x 8' throughout. But it can be helpful and gives a quick overview; an advantage, when the music has an irregular structure.

Analysis and notation can be either simpler or more detailed than the above suggests:
1) Just note A B C, verse, chorus and interlude respectively (see page 75).
2) The music can be counted and analyzed beat by beat (see page 176); for every beat or measure you note characteristics and create the choreography for this – or you can work intuitively.

Tip: Give each eight-count (2 x 4/4) a number to keep track or refer to, e.g. if you make notes for dancers.

Dance Fitness Training

Music	Beats/time	Choreography (basis)
	4 x 8 (0:00) B Freak	Stand hips STS, arms UD in front of the torso: R 4, L 4, B 8
	4 x 8 (0:18) A Have...	R Pivot ¼ turn walk 2, 4. Mambo, pivot 1/1, stand, torso D/U
	4 x 8 (0:34) A Young.	L Pivot ¼ turn walk 2, 4. Mambo, pivot 1/1, stand, shake hips 8.
	2 x 8 (0:50) B Freak	Jump O, arms O, stand shake body, 1-4. Jump I, arms cross by chest, 5-8. 2.
	4 x 8 (0:59) A All ...	R Pivot ¼ turn walk 2, 4. Mambo, pivot 1/1, stand body D/U
Chic:	4 x 8 (1:14) A Night...	L Pivot ¼ turn walk 2, 4. Mambo, pivot 1/1, stand shake hips 8.
Le Freak	2 x 8 (1:30) B Freak	Jump O, arms O, stand shake body, 1-4. Jump I, arms cross by chest, 5-8. 2.
3:34	4 x 8 (1:38) C v Now	Jump/hop STS (turn ½) 3, twist. 4
BPM	4 x 8 (1:54) C i	Step touch 8, ST R2 L2, 2. Move hips into the movement.
120	4 x 8 (2:10) C v I say	Walk badkwards R 3, turn '4', wave. Walk backwards L 3, turn '8', wave. 4
	4 x 8 (2:26) C v Now	Jump/hop STS (turn ½) 3, twist. 4
	4 x 8 (2:42) A All ...	R Pivot ¼ turn walk 2, 4. Mambo, pivot 1/1, stand body D/U
	4 x 8 (2:59) A Night	L Pivot ¼ turn walk 2, 4. Mambo, pivot 1/1, stand shake hips 8
	4 x 8 (3:16) B Freak	Jump O, arms O, stand shake body, 1-4. Jump I, arms cross by chest, 5-8. 2. Walk, shake your body, 16.

Dance Fitness Show

Yello: Resistor. Analysis (first minute) and initial choreography notes.

TID	8-TAKT	MUSIKSTRUKTUR	BEN-/KROPSBEVÆGELSE	ARMBEVÆGELSE	FORMATION
0:00	0			ARME UP HÆNDER RØRER	
	1		LIG PÅ RYG PÅ GULV →	HINANDEN 'BØLGE' 0±1	
	2			ARME O HOVED 1-4, OM PÅ NAVE	
	3			PRES KROP BAGUD	
	4		RUL OP OG STÅ RET RYGGEN MOD CENTER	RUL OP OG STÅ, ARME NED	
0:16	5		HOP 1KHB 14 H HOP VEND 14 H	ARME IND TIL KROP	
	6		HOP HOP 12 m H		
	7	FJERN SNAK I HØJTALER	HOP 12m H HOP 14 MOD	PÅ '5' SÆT H HÅND BAG ØRE	
	8	SNAK SNAK	GÅ LANGSOMT I TRIO'ER	KIG OP, LYTTENDE	
0:27	9	ORGEL	I BALANCE LØFT V BEN (-4), FØR H. ARM BAGUD (-8)	BEGGE ARME FREM I TRIO CENTRUM	
	10		H. ARM F (1-4) OP FRA BAL. (5-8)		
	11		DREJ 12 BACLENS V. OM MARKER BØJ NED MEJ	V. ARM TREKKER N/O BG ARME N/O	FLYT PLADS
	12		2. 'SLIDE' S.T. SLOW m 12 VENDING		
	13		STÅ -	ARME OPPEFRA NED OG HÆNDER PÅ HOVED	
	14	SKRT	STÅ + HURTIGE LØBERIN	RYST PÅ HOVED	
0:45	15	HURTIGE BÆKKENSLAG	LØB 8 UDAD VÆK FRA CENTRUM	FINGRE/ OPPEFRA ARME RYSTER OG NED	
	16	I SIDSTE SAMME	SPARK H/V BEN UD DREJ 12 H AJ LØB H/VH		
	17		SPARK F IND MOD/MIDTE P		
	18		KNÆLØFT H/V HIGH K, KNÆLØFT PÅ LINER		
0:57	19	7 SYNTH 'TÅGEHORN' FALDENDE	TRE OG TRE /TRIO LØBER 12 H	RØR/ STØT HINANDEN	
	20		2 SKILØB AJ ('5') 2 F/1B+2B/1F, 2 HOP, PÅ LINIE	GIV SLIP	
	21		2 SKILØB 2B/1F+2F/1B, 2 HOP, PÅ LINIE		
	22		TRE OG TRE /TRIO LØBER 12 V	RØR/ STØT HINANDEN	
	23	'GO'	GÅ/TRAMP 2 GÅ UD I (4) NY FORMA-TION: GÅ I STILLING 2 PÅ STED	PÅ 8 -OG - HOP OP/STÅ ARME OP	

176

About the author

Marina Aagaard, Master of Fitness and Exercise, and part-time associate professor of sports specializing in fitness, dance and bodily expressions.

She is former national coach of AER gymnastics and consultant and course instructor for the Danish Gymnastics Federation and Sports Confederation of Denmark in charge of education, conventions, courses and development from 1995-2008.

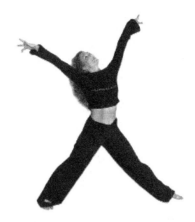

Before that, Marina was regional manager of aerobics and health club manager for the health club chain Form og Figur, 1990-1991, and managing director of the family health club BodyTeria, 1991-1999. At the same time Marina have been busy at her company aagaard as a lecturer and consultant for many different organisations.

Marina has written numerous articles on health and fitness for newspapers and magazines. She is author of a series of fitness bestsellers.

Marina is a certified Holistic Lifestyle Coach, CHEK Institute, and a certified aerobics instructor and personal trainer (gold), by ACE.

During the 90's she worked as a Master Trainer, Step/Slide Reebok. In 1993-1994 she starred in the Eurosport Step Reebok series with Gin Miller, the inventor of step.

Later on Marina had her own morning-TV fitness show for a two-year period.
As a choreographer Marina created several shows for national television, DR, dance and fitness programmes.

Marinas interest in elite training and performance lead to judging activity within the IAF, NAC and FISAF. She went on to serve as a juge breveté, a.o. difficulty judge, in AER gymnastics for the Federation Internationale de Gymnastique, FIG, and judged at every EC, WC and World Cerico final from 1995-2004.

Marina lives with her husband architect Henrik Elstrup in the bay area Kaloe Vig, Jutland, Denmark. Her interests are fitness and wellness, running, skiing and skating, arts, music, dance, nature, travelling and cars.

FITNESS BOOKS

Stability Ball Exercises
Fitness and Performance Exercises for
Strength, Stability and Flexibility
274 pages

A comprehensive compilation of stability ball
exercises. Over 450 exercises with the stability
ball, also know as the Swiss ball or strength
ball. Plus even more variations.
One-on-one, partner and group exercises
at all levels, for beginners, intermediate and
advanced exercisers, including elite athletes.
With more than 900 photos and step-by-step
text on proper exercise technique. And a guide
to progressing ball exercises.
As a unique feature the book includes the most
effective and enjoyable warm-up/cardio and
stretching exercises with the ball.
Stability Ball Exercises, is a valuable reference
book for any coach, trainer, physical exercise
leader, personal trainer, physiotherapist, group
exercise instructor, and PE teacher.

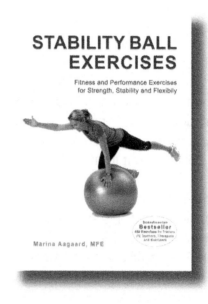

Resistance Training Exercises
Fitness and Performance Exercises for
Strength, Stability and Mobility
290 pages

A comprehensive compilation of resistance
training exercises; over 500; bodyweight,
dumbbells, barbells, tubes, bands and balls.
For one-on-one, partner and group strength
training at all levels, beginners, intermediate and
advanced. With more than 1000 photos and
step-by-step text on exercise technique, basic
posture, starting position, safety precautions.
The book features basic, intermediate as well as
advanced exercises from top to toe, from inner
unit to outer unit, for optimal health, fitness and
performance and fun, time-efficient workouts.
Including multi-level partner exercises.
Resistance Training Exercises, is a valuable
reference book for any coach, trainer, physical
exercise leader, personal trainer, group exercise
instructor, physiotherapist and PE teacher.

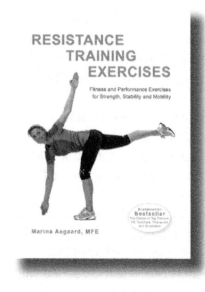

Lightning Source UK Ltd.
Milton Keynes UK
UKOW07f1122080817
306906UK00004B/106/P